Nursing School

School

A Nursing Student's Comprehensive Guide of Tips

(The Information You Need to Know Before Starting Nursing School)

Curt Deshields

Published By **John Kembrey**

Curt Deshields

Nursing School: A Nursing Student's Comprehensive Guide of Tips (The Information You Need to Know Before Starting Nursing School)

ISBN **978-1-7782615-9-6**

No part of this guidebook shall be reproduced in any form without permission in writing from the publisher except in the case of brief quotations embodied in critical articles or reviews.

Legal & Disclaimer

The information contained in this book is not designed to replace or take the place of any form of medicine or professional medical advice. The information in this book has been provided for educational & entertainment purposes only.

The information contained in this book has been compiled from sources deemed reliable, and it is accurate to the best of the Author's knowledge; however, the Author cannot guarantee its accuracy and validity and cannot be held liable for any errors or omissions. Changes are periodically made to this book. You must consult your doctor or get professional medical advice before using any of the suggested remedies, techniques, or information in this book.

Table Of Contents

Chapter 1: the importance of self-care

The nursing school experience can be intimidating! This is a unique environment similar to any other. It helps prepare future registered nurses for the many challenges they'll face during their professional lives. Nursing is an extremely demanding profession that requires professionals to be on their guard. It is a difficult and demanding environment. The school not only prepares students for the challenges they will likely encounter in the near coming years, but it also prepares them for the demands of their long work hours and plans. The nursing school grinds students down that when they are done with their degree, they've gained enough information about what to anticipate from their future career, and the strength needed to tackle the challenges.

A nursing education can test you in a variety of methods. However, this isn't a reason to be scared or discouraged. It is essential to have a survival kit - a tool that can help to prepare and anticipate the physical and mental issues of attending nursing school. This book provides that source with a step-by -step "how to survive nursing school" book that can make the idea of nursing school an easier task.

CHARITY BEGINS AT HOME

Nursing staff care for patients. The primary responsibility of nurses is to provide proper medical health care and to provide comfort for patients suffering from illness or unable to provide for themselves. This is an essential capability that could frequently make the difference in the outcome of a situation that could be life or death. Making someone ready for the job takes a lot of effort. Thus, nursing schools come with extensive curriculums and rigid study plan. If students find themselves in the demands of this type of atmosphere, they try the best they can to handle the stress of their job and neglect the most crucial aspect, which is providing for themselves.

When you work in this type of environment, self-care is essential. Self-care is the essential tool that is that is available to each nursing student who needs to manage their hectic studying and working program. Untreated self-care leads to severe difficulties in managing massive workloads. It's important to keep in mind that giving back starts in the home. That is, if you are tasked with providing health care, the primary patient to benefit from this care must be yourself. There is no way to expect you to provide care for another in the event that you're not adequately taken care of yourself.

It is important to remember that a good night's sleeping is vital for your body to function. Everyone needs at least eight hours of rest every throughout the day. If you're a person who uses a lot of effort each day - whether physically or mentally demanding, they need to rest even more. Consider your body as a piece of machinery that requires maintenance every day to function properly. A healthy diet and a sufficient quantity of rest are the things your body requires to replenish its strength and energy to function later. In the end, sleep deprivation can cause an energy deficit or extreme fatigue. It can also lead to sometimes even disease. Don't compromise having enough sleep!

A small amount of training can be beneficial for your health. It will help keep your body in shape and keep your mind sharp. This will allow you to keep away from fatigue, and will ensure that you are in top shape to be able to tackle your exhausting work and studying time with renewed enthusiasm each time. It doesn't necessarily suggest that you should go to the gym full effort and work on chiseled muscles or abs on a washboard. It's just a gentle aerobic workout to stay well. Regular physical exercise, when coupled with a demanding work routine could make the body weak, leaving it more susceptible to suffering. A gentle workout or simply a stroll outdoors in fresh air can help you stay healthy. In addition, it's the perfect stress-buster as well as it helps to prevent ailments and keep you physically active.

Don't underestimate the benefits in drinking water. An exhausting routine will cause you to become dehydrated, especially when you reside in a warmer environment. The body fluids are released via sweat. Make sure you stay watered and drink lots of fluids. Each person is different in their water needs according to their gender and size, age and lifestyle, however given your chaotic and fast-paced lifestyle it is essential to drink a minimum of at minimum one gallon of water each daily. It isn't just for quenching your thirst, it's also vital for all processes in your body. Drinking water should be consumed regularly throughout the day in order to prevent becoming dehydrated.

In class, you'll be taught how to create a balanced diet, which is the first step to an active and healthy lifestyle. Learn why it's crucial to eat well if the body is going to operate optimally, and then implement this knowledge to your own life too. As nurses You'll have to educate your patients of the importance in a healthy diet and the benefits of it, and how it keeps their bodies healthy, active and engaged. Thus, you should follow through with what you say and implement the idea of a balanced and healthy diet for you. The exercise, the sleep and every other method aren't as effective without adequate diet.

Make sure you eat a balanced, healthy diet that will allow you to manage the hectic working schedule you're expected to encounter during nursing school. If you're eating poorly and aren't well-nourished, you'll not have enough energy and strength to succeed. Thus, it's important to pay attention to the food you eat and make sure you consume enough food and you keep a healthy diet. It is a job that involves you caring for others and relies on being physically and mentally healthy.

MAINTAIN A HEALTHY BALANCE

It's rather ironic that the majority of students entering nursing school suffer from physical or mental stress as a result of stress caused from the arduous work load throughout the course. The primary job of a nurse is to safeguard the well-being and health of other people, however, it is surprising that nursing students are prone to neglect to follow the same guidelines for well-being in their personal lives. The result could be that several of them being susceptible to disorders like fatigue, depression or minor ailments, as well as at times, even nervous breaks. Do not let anxiety get you down! Maintaining your fitness and health is the most important factor in getting through every challenge of the nursing program.

Many nursing students don't know the importance of being able to find a balanced equilibrium between their studies and leisure to ensure that they don't have negative impacts to their physical and mental wellbeing. Stress can take a heavy toll on the body as well as the mind. And if we allow it to overwhelm us and take over it can create an array of issues for our own health. Stress can cause anxiety and exhaustion and can trigger feelings of loneliness and depression and eventually cause more serious illnesses.

If you're always exhausted and exhausted, it will be difficult concentrate in classes or dedicate enough time to study. In the end, your academic performance is likely to fall. Given the sheer amount of work you must do at nursing schools and the longer you're sick you are sick, the more your academic performance will suffer. It is sometimes more beneficial to stop and stop for a breather and unwind. Health is a top priority; this is the message that nurses receive.

Chapter 2: Study Strategies

Once you have realized how important it is to maintain a healthy and effective care plan for your self and have a few ideas about how you can achieve the right balance within the midst of a hectic lifestyle The next thing to focus on is in a systematic approach to studying. The curriculum for nursing schools is both extensive and technically demanding. The same is true for medical schools. To maximise your ability to get the most value of your time studying You must find an effective study method. It is essential to have a regular and efficient method of conducting your education if you are hoping to be successful within any curriculum that is medically focused.

TO EACH THEIR OWN

Today, the Internet as well as self-help studies guides provide you with an endless range of ways to solve the problems you face with studying. It is easy to find an array of creative methods for studying, all claim to aid in studying and perform better on examinations. The guides explain the advantages and cons of every method and usually include professional testimonies. However, the reality is very different. The best method is not the same for everybody and you have to determine which method will work best for you. Consider teachers in the classroom who are experts in a variety of topics and frequently vary on their style of teaching and methods. They have a unique approach to their subject matter. They utilize a range of strategies and techniques, particularly those that fit their particular area of specialization. Students should also apply the same method when choosing which method of study works most effectively for them.

Imagine you're enrolling in two classes: one course that is designed to help to understand the treatment of people who have mental health issues as well as another that is focused on nutrition. They differ greatly in terms of content and method and therefore it's important to address each independently. The same study plan doesn't always be effective for all of them on the same basis. First, you must examine your strengths and areas of weakness. Maybe you're great at remembering information, but not so good at communicating or writing down specific answers. In the same way, you might be a good student in practical or practical classes, but you're not as well with the theoretical aspect. When you've come up with an outline that outlines your weaknesses and strengths you'll be in better position to choose the best method for you, in every circumstance.

LET GO OF PRECONCEIVED NOTIONS

Everyone will advise you on what to do and how you should proceed with your studies. In most cases it is a good thing to have well-meaning relatives and friends they are simply worried about the workload you face and are eager to provide support. Be aware of their advice But remember that choosing what is the most effective approach typically involves firsthand knowledge, and it is you who are the most accurate person to judge what you are good at and weak in, and of the approach which is right for you.

There are a variety of methods that to study. Most people make use of flashcards or develop quizzes using the content of the class. Think about creating interesting acronyms using medical terminology, or include the difficult medical terminology into songs that are fun and will help you remember them. Discover what is natural to you. This will aid in making studying more enjoyable.

Get rid of any assumptions and biases you've had and pick a program that is right for you, not necessarily one that is suited to all of the general populace. What is important is that you're completely at ease with the way you do your research.

FOCUS, FOCUS, FOCUS!

The right approach and method for learning is just the start. The system will enable you to learn better and more effectively, but, ultimately you will need to learn. This will not be an easy course but it will be challenging and test you on every step of the process. You have to put into everything your best with total dedication and complete concentration. It's not just about learning to pass your examinations and earn good marks. The lessons you'll learn in the end will have more than just that. In the course of your professional career, you'll get the chance to use your learning in real-world situations and help ease some suffering, or perhaps even help save lives. Learn what you're trained to be very serious, and not only as a result of an excellent score.

Staying with the system of study that is effective for you and being able quickly gather and remember data from every corner of the medical spectrum will not just help you prepare to pass the exams and score excellent grades, it can also help you gain knowledge about the subject. The knowledge gained and the presence of mind can be useful when it comes to life or death situations, and will help many patients in the many years to in the future. It's never too late to begin preparing for those. Learning and retaining all of the information is a major challenge. All you need is focus and discipline. concentration.

If you've got a solid method of studying with the proper concentration, you've achieved a lot. When you've decided what you want to do with your study and how to organize your time, it is important to establish positive and healthy habits. It will help you adhere to the method you've adopted, and enable you to make the most effective utilization of the program and the methods it employs. Setting up a study plan is the very first step to the long-distance trip. The actual journey lies before you. only you've packed your luggage and made journey arrangements.

ORGANIZATION IS KEY

There's nothing like a perfect system. Being organized is the first stage in developing effective studying practices. Nursing school's curriculum is incredibly extensive and varied that it's very easy to become lost when you're trying to figure it out. A lot of times, students don't have a clue where to begin. They often resort to random, unorganized studying. This can do more harm than beneficial. If you want to increase the potential of your studies, organize your study method.

The very first thing you'll need is a Wall calendar that you will be able to view at any time. Begin by marking significant dates associated with the course in question. Note your exams dates, deadlines for assignments and tasks, in addition to any other important dates or deadlines to be remembered. The calendar can serve as a reference to keep you on track while reminding of obligations on a daily as well as a weekly and monthly basis. Reminding yourself of the deadline is the most effective and efficient method to make sure you achieve the deadline. It's true that we often get lax in our college lives. If we don't get informed that the deadline is less than forty-eight days away, it's possible that we won't even begin making progress on the task. To make the most of the excellent system you have created for studying You need to be organized to be successful. For it, a wall calendar can be extremely useful.

This calendar is helpful for in a macro-level but you'll also require an organized daily schedule. It can be accomplished with an electronic or manual organizer with a list of your day-to-day tasks. Although it may appear to be something unnecessary or for you however, whenever you're facing the challenge of finishing several tasks, assignments, or lessons in the shortest time and you're not sure how to organize your time, it's important to keep a schedule which will help keep you on track and make sure you don't let your academics or your health suffer. With the advent of technology there's no need for any additional calendars. The smartphone can handle perfectly. The majority of smartphones have a lot of intelligence, and are smarter than what we're used to! They're a fantastic method to stay up to date and on top of our daily routine.

Many books and guides will provide you with tips regarding how to organize your life. Don't be shy or reluctant to search for them and ask for help if you'll locate it. There's no doubt you'll require all the support that you get. Every major school of nursing across the country offer the facilities to help students and teachers. They are excellent resources for students as they assist students in becoming more efficient in how they manage their time at the school. They can help you create efficient study methods as well as find more efficient methods to adhere to your plan. If your institution offers one of these centers and you are interested, take advantage of it. This will relieve a great deal of your burden from your shoulders, aiding in easing the studying burden.

DEVELOP GOOD STUDY HABITS

My mom would always tell her children to establish good ways of living. When I think at my past, I can see that she was right. Of course, moms are right on these things. The use of a schedule can assist with organizing your thoughts as well as creating a structure and schedule for studying. In the end it is necessary to establish the right habits for studying for the system to work.

A lot of students like to review and study lectures prior to the class. This will allow you to know the subject matter of your lecture as well as giving you advantages in the sense that you'll know more since you'll already be knowledgeable about the topic that you are studying. This helps you focus more effectively, and will help make the class much more engaging. If we're engaged in what is being taught We have better retention and retention. In order to further enhance your learning experience You can go over the subjects that are being taught during class in an hour of your lecture. Research suggests that recall is most effective within the first 24 hours after learning something unfamiliar. Repetition of subjects within this period helps us retain the information for a more extended period of time, usually some weeks. By doing this it will help you learn and retain more information, thereby maximising your knowledge in the class while also making the most of you time in the most effective manner that you can.

Studies have proven scientifically that the most optimal timing to be studying is in the morning, or later in the evening. There is a greater amount of quiet in these hours. This is dependent on the individual in determining the best time for their needs. For some, it might be difficult to wake up early to do their homework, whereas others may become exhausted when night comes in. Select a time which suits your personal needs and will allow you to concentrate free of distractions and interruptions.

Chapter 3: Study Groups

Although studying on your own can be beneficial, the idea of forming an academic group is mandatory in nursing schools. Nursing schools are unlike other educational program since the very first class of students you meet at the time of registering will probably be the same people you'll be with throughout your course. The single aspect that sets the nursing program distinct. It is always a good idea to mix with others and build acquaintances early. Everyone needs friendships for emotional assistance. But what we tend to overlook is that our friends are also a great help when we are in a state of academic hazard. It is common to select among our closest friends individuals who are on the same page with us and who we feel comfortable with and are able to count on. If the people you are friends with are studying in the same class as us, then nothing could make more sense to join an academic group and benefit from each others' expertise in forming effective studying habits.

BENEFITS OF STUDY GROUPS

A well-organized study group has the capacity to aid students improve their academic performance. Helps students to overcome academic problems by offering these advantages:

Goodbye to Procrastination--Study groups are known for one great feature: they meet at regular times and for a fixed number of hours. In the end, there's no place for the procrastination. When you study in a group that is well-organized all members keep an eye on each other and make sure that one isn't a member regularly. If we're on our own at home, we are able to not study until the last moment. If we're in a group, it's important to are required to attend in a specified time, and continue to work for the entire duration of the gathering. Study groups create an orderly method.

When students study together learning happens more quickly as opposed to studying on your own. It is mainly because of the fact that when you study together it is easier for the group to be better in all subjects. If you're stuck on an issue and need help, the members of your study group can help as well as help you save time trying to solve the puzzle on your own.

"Seeing Things from an entirely new perspective. We all view the world from a different viewpoint. Most of the time, it's hard to get out of the box and view the world in a fresh light. Study groups can help you attain that viewpoint academically. Through gaining new perspective about a particular subject You can appreciate many new perspectives and learn differently.

Learn New Study Skills - Every student develops their own system and methods of studying. In groups, when you study and interact with fellow students to learn their strategies as well as learning methods. This will help you discover an approach or strategy which is suited to your style of learning and preferences. Compare the advantages and disadvantages of every technique and you'll see that studying groups teach you so much more than the basics.

An Innovative Approach to Studying Alone can become a tedious exercise, but studying groups are a great way to break the routine. As the group when you get bored and boring, there is no need to stop doing your homework. Instead, you can take the choice of discussing the topic in a group discussion with your fellow classmates. It is a great way to break the monotony, and refresh your brain, yet not interfere with the process of learning. There are some people who cannot be able to study for hours in silence. In these cases, study group discussions are particularly helpful.

There is no room for gaps in studies, you get the chance to review your notes with fellow students and evaluate the quality of your notes. You can also correct any mistakes you may have as well as get suggestions to improve your note-taking. It is important to eliminate gaps which could interfere with the learning process. Study group's collective learning generally covers every topic in the syllabus. So, you'll most likely be able to cover everything.

HOW TO GO ABOUT IT

Study groups are fantastic! Be aware, however it isn't the case that every group can be regarded as a great study group. Choose your study partners with care and meet the study objectives within the group in order so that it is worthwhile. An effective study group is the ideal method to exchange ideas and share knowledge. Make sure that your discussion does not diverge beyond the subject matter of study to routine chatter in the classroom. It is essential to keep the focus when you are in a study class. It is essential to ensure that you reap the greatest benefits from the study group, so you can see the value for the organization. In the event that it doesn't, it will be a massive wasted of effort and time. These are some tips to help make your study group more efficient:

1. A study group needs to be small and not comprise more than five participants. This

ensures that the strengths and flaws of each participant's strengths complement one others, as well as ensuring to ensure that the group doesn't transform into a gossip shack. Also, this improves the efficacy and efficiency for the entire group.

2. Create specific goals for the group, in the same manner that you establish objectives for yourself in your studies. Each meeting should meet those goals. Only this way can the group achieve success.

3. Study groups are a team effort. The group leader should be the one who takes the initiative, but do not let it transform into a solo show. The goal is to learn through collaboration. Everyone should participate equally in the sharing and learning procedure.

4. Study groups don't replacement for personal learning, they're a complement to it. It is essential to find an equilibrium between these two. If you can do this then, learning is much more enjoyable because of it.

Chapter 4: Success in the Classroom

The time spent in the classroom is an crucial element in the nursing curriculum. The majority of programs are split into multiple semesters, each comprising multiple courses that need the use of a specific duration of time that includes the theory as well as clinical tasks. Students study the theory within the classroom. The theory forms the basis for all subsequent information gained from clinical practice. Therefore, it is crucial, and the classes are essential. It is equally crucial to have clinical hours in that they enable students to use their theoretical understanding in the practice. In combination, theoretical and clinical skills are the basis of the nursing curriculum.

The importance of the classroom is vital and that you need to pay attention. If you don't pay attention during classes, you can are putting more pressure on yourself later on. If you are attentive in the class, you stand greater chances of grasping the concept and how they are taught. This will make a difference in the amount of work in the future.

BE INQUISITIVE

Don't forget that you're a student! However straightforward or unimportant the topic could seem to you or how proficiently your professor is teaching it, there will always be a thing that's going to leave you confused. There could be a complicated method or concept which isn't clear for the person who is reading it. Be sure to ask questions in order to clarify any confusion that you may be having. A lot of students hesitate to pose questions to students for fear of being embarrassed. This should be the least of your concerns! You can ask for help - it's only a sign of your concentration, as well as the desire to answer any questions.

Most students like to talk about questions with colleagues after class instead of asking their instructor. They could be able of clarifying details to a certain extent; but no explanation is more effective than one given by a professional who is familiar with this subject matter for years. The professor is more qualified to address your concerns. Therefore, if you've got concerns or questions, don't be afraid to ask your instructor. The professors are always happy to address these concerns!

"Curiosity killed the cat"? Don't you want to play the cat. You'd rather be considered"top dog" instead "top dog" instead. In order to achieve that it is essential to be interested. If there's anything you learn during the course or in a class that you aren't understanding then inquire. The clinical courses are essential because they provide you with skills that stay in your mind for the rest of time, abilities which could save lives later. If you are unsure about an exact procedure, you can request the instructor to explain the procedure, or describe it in a simpler way. It is important to remember that the purpose of your professor is to teach you. They will be happy to help you to clear any questions. If your professor is unable to help due to limitations in time or for any other motive, you can approach the instructor during class for a date to explain the process to you. Make the effort and become on top of your studies!

PRACTICE MAKES PERFECT

Through the course there is a chance that you'll encounter some new concepts and practices. You will discover a lot of interesting things you will discover. The most difficult thing is to retain every bit of information over the course of time. Therefore, make the effort to master and grasp all new concepts and techniques accurately. There must be no space for uncertainty. If you are in doubt, discuss the doubts with your instructor or your professor.

You'll need to work at it lots. Repetition the procedure every day until you're the Zen expert in handling these procedures. You must be skilled with the techniques so that you're confident about performing the correct way, and not messing around without any guidance. This is what learning about a process signifies! Practical experience can help you implement the theoretical information and you will not be able to do that without enough experience.

INTERACTIONS WITH UPPERCLASSMEN

When you are at the school you will interact with three types of individuals throughout the school year you are with: your fellow students as well as your teachers and the upperclassmen. This article has discussed how your interactions between the two are expected to be. Let's discuss how you interact with the upperclassmen. The environment of nursing schools differs from the typical college setting in many different ways. One of the more striking distinctions is the absence of any clear hierarchical distinctions. Your classmates are likely to be very friendly and accommodating individuals who will be able to assist you in your quest to become a guidance throughout the course. Create a healthy and positive connection with your upperclassmen and engage with them. They're more knowledgeable with managing the syllabus, teachers, and the tests. Their understanding of these matters can be invaluable.

SENIORS: THE SAVIORS

Some people believe that even though the seniors may have of experience and are able to know more about their program and school but their expertise is fading relative to instructors and other employees. There is also a belief that teachers will always have your best interests to be in the forefront and senior class may not have an ideal influence. The truth is in the theory, however life isn't all about theory. It's not always clear and never straightforward. While professors may have an explanation that is more thorough and more about specific topics related to the program but interaction with senior students is more of an informal basis. However friendly your professor might be you are still their instructor and some students may feel uncomfortable approaching their professors, and the interaction may be more formal. Students who are older can be more approachable and are able to overcome the rift that may be separating a student from their instructor.

Seniors are often the sources for advice that is needed during the stressful atmosphere of nursing school. However they may act as acquaintances and not be seen in the role of authoritative people. They've experienced and seen all the things you'll go through. They are aware of how to handle the curriculum in nursing school. In reality, there will be individual variations. Let it serve as a source of information to you. Decide on other aspects based on your personal experiences. The advice you receive doesn't necessarily mean that you will learn the entire nursing school survival skills. While you're going through the curriculum, you'll have to learn a few things on your own.

Seniors can supply the information you need, such as how a certain professor's method of teaching works and how he/she they prefer assignments to be done. They can provide you with an understanding of what are likely to encounter in a course or class, as well as from your entire course. Make sure to take in as much knowledge as you can. It can help in making it easier to endure the demands of nursing school.

THE MENTOR PROGRAM

There are nursing schools that have mentoring programs, which include the relationship between professors and peers. The program permits the mentors to share their knowledge to the students and aid students overcome the obstacles and challenges they encounter within the course. It is the role of the mentor to support the student's development academically, with a focus on course and performance in the classroom. They are an advisor who can help the student to navigate the unfamiliar terrain of college.

These programs assist the student to adjust to the new environment. Mentors for students are selected based on their ability to communicate, trust, and interpersonal abilities, with their trustworthiness. Mentoring is known to assist students to adjust to the unfamiliar environment faster. This is especially beneficial in nursing schools, as the curriculum is so extensive that the students who are new have little time to get used to the new environment. Mentors can serve as a role model to young students not just through their guidance, however, they also assist them as they progress.

Peer mentoring can be described as individual peer mentorship, group seminars about topics such as organizational and managing time, new and prospective student orientations discussions in nursing introductory classes, and handouts with information about topics that are important to nurses. A major advantage of having a mentor system is that it not just helps to improve the academic performance of those who are just beginning their studies however it also improves social connections. Mentors and mentees are able to create friendships that last for an entire lifetime. It is always beneficial having a mentor you can trust in this difficult situation. Peer mentorship has been utilized extensively in the education of healthcare workers. This kind of help is offered by volunteers nurses and nursing alumni as well as seniors.

The main benefit of this course that students are prone to overlook is the fact that it establishes the concept of a student nurse network within the school which allows students to work together in order to accomplish their objectives and assist them in overcoming the issues they face. It also sets the scene for their future as they are asked to cooperate with one and work together.

It is true that mentors are usually overlooked, but the value their advice is more than many people believe. Within every college setting, you will find a variety of little things such as book-related handouts to notes from class and advice which can only be obtained from a single source - someone that is ahead on the course.

GET TO KNOW YOUR PROFESSORS

Professors play a major role in the course of college. They serve as your guide, mentors or, sometimes, your close friends. A good teacher and the ability to build a strong rapport with them could be a boon for your success during your time in nursing college.

Chapter 5: Making the Most of a Break

Breaks are a period when you are able to take a break from the craziness of school. You can take a moment to relax, and simultaneously locating ways outside the course to enhance and continue your knowledge. One of the biggest mistakes that students make is that they do not use the time they have off productively, and disrupting their studies. A lot of students take classes on breaks. They are however, generally not the case. It is important to remember that taking a break from your prescribed school schedule is not time to be devoted to trivial activities. Instead, use it to acquire experience that is relevant to the subject you are studying.

Learning is one of the aspects of nursing school that has to continue. In the event of a break or not the process of learning should not stop. There are many possibilities for enhancing your knowledge when you are on break. You could consider a part-time or daily work at the local hospital or clinic. The position of a nursing assistant can make you money as well as help you prepare for a clinical environment. When you are completing your education the main focus must always be your studies.

THE AIDE FACTOR

An opportunity to work as a nurse assistant at a local hospital or clinic can assist in offering you more clinical experiences that help you prepare for the practical aspects of your profession as a nurse. It's a fantastic opportunity to make the most of your vacation time. This will allow you to apply what you learned from the classroom and during clinical classes in a professional environment. It will allow you to observe daily tasks in nursing, and also learn manage multiple patient cases at once. This is an excellent learning experience that helps students move from college to work. It could also help you gain a foothold on the path to an employment opportunity in the future. This can be a fantastic chance to network in your field. It is an excellent opportunity to join and expand your circle of professionals.

They don't know the value they can benefit from these experiences when developing a career in nursing. If you're a person with a love in nursing, this could be the ideal way to acquire the real-world knowledge.

LOOKING BACK AND FORWARD, TOO

An opportunity to work as a nursing aid during summer vacation helps you to develop new abilities and gain experience. However, don't forget everything you've learned in your classroom. The summer break gives ample time to review and refresh your skills. It is important to make sure that your knowledge isn't lost when examinations are finished. In the end, as we've mentioned before it's not just about doing your best to get a grade, but you're also trying to develop skills that can assist you in saving life in the future. It is important to keep this information for a lengthy period of time. No matter how much you have studied and you're done with them, don't just sit and unwind!

If you feel it's too difficult for you, do not be concerned. There's always the possibility to look in the future. You can, for instance, go through the textbooks of the coming classes. This can be done along with other jobs that or other job you hold. It shouldn't be a problem, and will provide you with confidence when the semester begins. You'll feel more at ease with your knowledge gained over the summer time off. If you're on an inclination to compete, you'll notice that you're a bit more advanced than your fellow students since you'll be well-versed in the subjects and ideas that are being taught in class making things a little simpler for the students.

By putting in a little effort you'll accomplish much by making life less stressful for you. Utilize your break time wisely!

PREPARATION FOR NCLEX

It is the NCLEX is the exam that is required to license nurses across the United States. The NCLEX-RN exam is an extensive examination that demands a large amount of studying time. The preparation to take your NCLEX (National Council Licensure Exam) by using a book to review is an excellent option to study subjects in nursing even during breaks. Be sure to take the NCLEX all through the course of your studies not only during the break.

The most important thing you can be able to do is try to manage your studies and your clinical classes to allow you to dedicate some time in preparation for your NCLEX. For this make sure you be using a high-quality NCLEX review guide, which can be used to help you prepare for each test. Completely completing NCLEX types of questions is among the most effective ways to prepare for the upcoming nursing examination and also for the NCLEX test. We'll take a look what NCLEX tests are, and the reason what they mean for the profession of nursing.

WHAT ARE THE NCLEX EXAMINATIONS?

The NCLEX exam is the standard to determine who is registered nurses across the United States. It is created and is owned through the National Council of State Boards of Nursing, Inc. (NCSBN). The NCSBN conducts the exam for its member board. It comprises nursing boards from all

50 states of the United States, as well as the District of Columbia, and the four U.S. territories, including American Samoa, Guam, Northern Mariana Islands, and Guam, Northern Mariana Islands, and the U.S. Virgin Islands.

The goal of these tests is to make sure that the nursing profession is of high quality and takes care of the sick within the United States so that there can be a proper safeguarding of the health of all Americans. These exams are designed to ensure quality standards within the field of nursing. Every board of nursing within the region or state requires each licensed candidate to pass the NCLEX-RN test for Registered Nurses. This exam has been designed to test the skills, knowledge, and capabilities that are crucial for the secure and efficient training of nurses at entry level.

It is important to keep in mind is NCLEX exam isn't focused on memorization neither is it a study of books. To be able to pass you must be aware of the notion that is behind the critical process. Since 2010, the NCLEX focused on the way students manage and prioritize their tasks.

The NCLEX exams are offered as computer-based adaptive testing (CAT) style. It is currently administered via Pearson VUE in their network of Pearson Professional Centers (PPC).

HOW THE NCLEX REVIEW BOOKS HELP

The NCLEX review books can be the most effective option to find exam preparation materials to pass the NCLEX exam and nursing tests. The purchase of the NCLEX review book earlier in your career can be the ideal option if you're trying to pass the test. Keep in mind the fact that it's never late to review and practice NCLEX-like questions. The NCLEX review guides break into sections which correspond to the subjects of study within your nursing education. Making sure you answer questions before taking each exam can aid in improving your exam-taking abilities and will help you to understand how to put into practice the concepts you've that you have learned in class. The process of completing NCLEX type questions is among the most effective ways to learn at nursing schools. This helps you become familiar with the format and structure of the tests. The more you take practice and the more confident you will be proficient in answering questions. Remember that becoming familiar with the manner in which questions are structured during these tests is among the most effective preparation tools available that will help you get through the test. There are a variety of choices to choose from for NCLEX study books from various publishing houses. The most well-known options are:

Lippincott's Q&A Review for NCLEX-RN

NCLEX-RN Questions & Answers Made Incredibly Easy!

Mosby's Comprehensive Review of Nursing for NCLEX-RN Examination

Saunders Comprehensive Review for the NCLEX-RN Examination

Davis's Q&A for the NCLEX-RN Examination

Mosby's Review Cards for the NCLEX-RN Examination

There are a variety of other review publications available and some are available as electronic books on the Internet. They will assist you to discover your weaknesses areas and strengths, and will give ideas to think about. Utilizing these study books even while in the school can have two benefits. One, you are able to request your teachers to clarify the subject or question. The second reason is that the nursing course has the exact same curriculum as the exam content so the course of your program can aid you in preparing for your exam.

It is recommended to use the NCLEX review guide to the fullest extent and do as much practice as you are able to. As many questions as you can, and do it slowly, but steadily you'll be closer to being able to pass the NCLEX test.

Chapter 6: Tools for Handling Stress

Nursing schools often put on a lot of pressure. This can be overwhelming students and cause stress in particular the newly graduated struggling to get used to the hectic work schedule. The overwhelming amount of work as well as the tight deadlines can significantly impact students in nursing negatively. Certain studies indicate that levels of stress experienced by nursing students are more than their peers in social work, medical as well as pharmacology.

The issue is exacerbated due to the fact that there are no more nursing students in the present young adults recently graduated from high school. In the last few years, this occupation is now attracting people looking to make a career transition in their 30s or 40s. They have also added to their families as needing to concentrate on their studies as well, they must take care of their spouses and kids. The situation can become very difficult. The nursing school experience isn't easy however, you've got the drive, determination and ability to conquer these obstacles and come out unscathed.

Let's examine how we will be able to face the challenging and turbulent times of nursing school, and keep the calmness we need to maintain.

SELF-BELIEF IS CRUCIAL

There is a saying that, even when you lose everyone around and you remain confident in yourself, no one can stop you. This may appear to be a film-like exaggeration However, it's actually real. Don't underestimate the importance in self-belief. It will help you climb up mountains. There will be times when things won't go as smoothly You're likely to confront obstacles. There will be days that are tougher and more demanding more than other days. You must not become frustrated or discouraged due to this. When your life needs more of you, make sure that you are ready to do an even greater amount. Do not take a backseat. Never lose hope. Don't give up.

A belief in you and the abilities you have is key ingredient to aid you in overcoming obstacles even the toughest of situations. Research has shown that at least one third of nursing students experience pressure in one form or another, to the degree that it could trigger mental health issues including anxiety and depression. The primary source of stress for students in nursing is the clinical setting. Patients are anxious during clinical training due to different reasons including a lack prior experience, the fear of making errors, challenging patients, anxiety about being questioned by faculty worried about giving patients inaccurate information or medicines as well as fear of damaging a patient. This can be a major factor in the confidence of nurses, especially in the case of nurses who are newer.

It is crucial to believe in what you've learned from the course and in your capabilities. Believe in yourself, and confidence that you're competent for this work. Then you'll have the confidence to complete your job with complete honesty and integrity. The confidence you have in your self is the most important factor to get out of difficult situations or situations where you are in type of uncertainty or doubt. It is possible that you are experiencing fear and anxiety due to the fact that you are trying something different at first, plus, because your health and well-being is based on your judgement. Be careful not to let the anxiousness turn into doubt or fear. Do not let it take the way of you and make you to doubt your capabilities. If you are able to be confident in your abilities and believe in yourself, the majority of your problems will disappear.

FALL BACK ON YOUR SUPPORT SYSTEM

Personally, I've witnessed that situations such as these can make people reconsider the decision they made to pursue this career. A high workload as well as their perception of their inability to handle the demands of nursing force a lot of students to believe that perhaps nursing isn't the best choice for their needs. In this situation you should take some time to take a breath and think. Make sure you remember the main motivation behind your decision to work as nurses at all. Examine that motivation in a long and arduous. If you've got a genuine love for nursing, you'll discover that nothing will stop the work you enjoy. Any issue is not big enough to deter you of your true passion.

Additionally, you'll have friends as well as a system of support that you can count on at times like these. Speak to them, and talk about your emotions with them. Do not let yourself feel alone at this point. There are many ways that words of encouragement and words of comfort can accomplish quite a lot even though they seem insignificant. They have healing properties which many people don't recognize. Speak to your family and friends, as well as people who are concerned about you, and soon will discover that the problem may be only in your head because of the increasing tension you're experiencing. If the problem has been real, you need to remember that any problem can only be the most difficult solution. Be aware of that, and nothing is going to seem too complicated anymore.

TALK TO FELLOW NURSES

One of the most common mistakes we make in dealing anxiety and feeling overwhelmed is that we think that we're by ourselves and believe that nobody can understand our state of mental state. The thing we often ignore is the fact there are nurses similar to us. Some likely are suffering through similar situations and facing similar problems. If you ever feel lonely and unnoticed, speak with your colleagues. When you talk about your issues with them then you'll realize that you don't have to be an overwhelming burden. Because many of your coworkers had similar issues previously They are who are best placed to help you through your situation.

The nursing staff you choose to work with must be the equivalent of your second family. It is important to be able talk about your troubles with them. Most of the time, they will offer the ideal solutions because they're familiar with the type of anxiety you're experiencing.

STRESS CAN GET TO ANYONE

If you're feeling overwhelmed or stressed from the nursing school isn't a sign that you're not capable academically or even mentally. Stress can be a problem for any person. All of us feel pressured by things at one point or another throughout their lives. It's part of our human nature. It's a fact of life. The key is to not let the worry consume our minds. Every college, but especially one with as much pressure and difficulty like nursing schools students are often dragged within the frantic pace of life which is paired with the hefty amount of work. Many of the top students quickly become overwhelmed. Being a successful student is nothing related to the capacity to deal with stress, and it's not necessary to believe that you're lacking some thing if you're overwhelmed. Everybody is stressed by the tense environment.

REMEMBER TO RELAX

A lot of students forget to take a break during nursing schools. The curriculum is extensive, and the load is immense however, relaxation may be one of the best ways to ease the anxiety and stress that develops due to all the work and academic circumstances. The schedule of nursing school is always intense, with a lot of hundred hours of classes in theory and clinical training, paired with work, assignments, as well as internships. It is important to not let the strain of your work load consume your mind. Some stress can be good for your health. Stress acts as a stimulant that helps you reach your goals and encouraging you to get stronger towards your objectives. It triggers an adrenaline surge throughout the body which increases the focus of our minds and improves performance. However, like everything else (exclude chocolate!) the stress response is healthy when it is moderately consumed!

HOW TO RELAX

There isn't a universal approach to help you manage anxiety. The individual's needs will vary and the circumstances. Certain techniques for relaxation can keep your from being overwhelmed and assist you in getting the most value from the college experience, academically professionally and socially.

It isn't often possible for students to have the space to enjoy a break when they're in a crowded atmosphere, so long periods of time spent on activities like yoga and aerobics as effective for stress reduction, isn't often an option. One way to make them part of your daily schedule is to divide these activities into manageable pieces. Another effective method to help relax during your time at nursing school are to give your self positive affirmations, putting down your thoughts that are negative, picturing the outcome, and then, while you're closed your eyes and for a couple of minutes, taking time to visualize yourself being relaxed. A healthy amount of hydration as well as short shoulders massages could be beneficial to help you achieve an unwinding state.

They are also simple to learn however, they have none of the side effects.

DON'T FORGET TO LAUGH

In the midst of a chaotic life is time to de-stress and let go of all the tension that comes with it. There is a point in time that you're able to let go of all the tasks and simply unwind. The only thing will always be there is your humor which you'll be able to count upon frequently in nursing training. It is always beneficial to view the positive side of things and keep a smile regardless of the circumstances.

Many people misunderstand the concept of humor, and see it as an escape from reality. People believe that if you laugh at your problems it is a way to get rid of the pain. It's not the case. When you see the positive aspect of your issues by focusing on the positive, you're building your confidence and getting ready to face the problem. If you can see the good side of challenges the situation becomes less daunting and the solution will become more clear. Do not think that embracing an occasional chuckle does not constitute a way to escape. In fact, it's a necessity when you're in a crisis. If you don't have a sense of laughter, you'll be dwelling on your sadness, which can make your issues worse and increase to the point of being even worse.

Laughter is the most effective solution to any problem. It's relaxing. It will help alleviate all kinds of issues almost instantly. In terms of science, it is possible to say that laughing releases endorphins into the brain similar to eating something that you like (think chocolate!). They are the substances that make us feel good inside our bodies, which make us feel positive and motivated. However, this doesn't mean laughing can solve all our issues or eliminate our troubles. But, it does provide an individual the confidence to tackle and overcome challenges more effectively. It boosts confidence in ourselves and keeps us from becoming overcome by the circumstances.

Chapter 7: Helpful Resources

It is essential to take advantage of all the useful resources offered by the nursing school to provide. The schools of today have a wealth of options to make your time simpler and more enjoyable. It's a wise, prudent option to use all of these resources, since they're all designed to help students just like you. A few of the more common sources a school could provide include:

Libraries

Tutoring Centers

Computer labs

Career Centers

Health and Counseling Centers

Financial services

Make use of these resources as they're designed specifically by your school with the requirements and needs of students studying nursing with in the forefront. They're specifically designed for nursing students and offer information to help you get answers to a lot of your queries. In particular, it's more beneficial to visit the college library that is in your campus instead of one in the downtown area, since the library at your college will have every book, journal as well as articles on your subject. It is rare to encounter the circumstance needing to use external resources.

THE LIBRARY

The library is the center of any academic institution. Particularly for nursing schools this is even more important since, within the field of medicine the students are required to search for past references frequently. The library that is well-stocked can be extremely beneficial for every student. The library at nursing schools consists of a variety of books arranged in accordance with a standard system one of that is known as the Library of Congress Classification System. Certain libraries also have circulation books, which are usually located behind the wall. Books for reference, that don't circulate, can also be found. Libraries today are increasingly making their online catalog accessible via the Internet as well as through the institution's network.

Additionally, the college library typically subscribes to print magazines and online full-text journals as well. As opposed to books, journals typically do not circulate. At some institutions, audiotapes, videotapes and CDs are available on borrowing.

Students may also conduct online searches for the medical literature using the software of libraries including CINAHL or Nursing Reference Center, which typically are accessible on the network of your college. At some schools, librarians conduct special educational workshops on the use of the databases for clinical research, which makes the job easier.

Personal computer (PCs) can be found almost all the time accessible to students at the library.

COMPUTER LABS

Computers are available at nursing schools in order to enhance learning as well as to aid in the instruction of students. The computer lab is equipped with distinct stations and access to various nurse software programs. There is usually software that can be used to prepare for the NCLEX-RN exam. Computers are linked to hospital's document system and to the Internet. Many colleges provide students access via remote to a variety of nursing software applications. At major universities, nursing software is accessible to students in classes and tasks, and also to help with remediation.

NURSING ARTS LAB

Certain nursing programs offer labs which simulate the environment of a clinical or hospital settings, training students for exposure in the clinical setting. In most cases, there is at least four beds in Nursing Arts Labs, which simulate patient care facilities that are equipped with various models, manikins as well as equipment. Students may make use of the facilities, however only with supervision. Some schools also offer the option of a simulation lab with low-fidelity. Skills labs are a skill-building experience that is an essential part of many nursing classes since it assists students acquire the expertise and skills required for effective delivery of care to clients.

GUIDANCE AND COUNSELING

Counseling facilities are among the most recent developments in nursing schools. Students experiencing personal difficulties including familial issues, depression or emotional tension, or academic problems have the option of contacting confidentially Counseling services through the Student Counseling Center to receive assistance in dealing problems. The program has become commonplace in nursing colleges across the nation, and each student has the right to have an assessment for their personal situation and is followed by counseling, recommendation to the right professionals, and follow-up support which ensure that the needs of the student are taken care of. According to the ethical guidelines for counselors and similar service, all conversations are completely private and confidential.

Apart from these the majority of colleges offer different features and services created to make the student's institution life more comfortable and easier. It is recommended that you make use of available resources when it is needed and with no hesitation. Be aware that these services can be used at any time to your advantage.

STAY INFORMED

Universities and colleges, particularly big ones that receive state support, frequently appear to be a solitary bureaucracy. The large nursing schools are stuffed with multiple processes, departments and committees, it's easy to lose yourself among the paperwork. It's crucial to stay in the middle of all that disarray and remain informed on the events happening in the surrounding area. Someone who is aware and knowledgeable will more likely to make the most of opportunities than people who don't know about their environment.

From the beginning it is essential to stay conscious of various issues. When it comes to registering classes or making an application for financial aid there are numerous dates and procedures to be aware of and you're responsible to keep track of them. Nobody can hold your hand or guide you through each step You'll have to complete all the work on yourself.

THE IMPORTANCE OF THE STUDENT HANDBOOK

The handbook of students at any institution is among the best and most reliable sources of information regarding the institution. You should take note of this important resource as it contains all the information necessary information about the policies and guidelines in addition to the different guidelines and deadlines of the college. Many of the top nursing colleges across the nation require their students to acknowledge that they've read and understand the contents of the handbook and they are bound by the rules and regulations in the handbook and understanding the consequence of any policy breach. A thorough review of the handbook essential. It's essential that you study the handbook carefully, and pay attention to all rules guidelines, procedures, and regulations and be able to comprehend them properly.

The handbook for students at nursing schools provides complete details on issues such as physical and emotional risks as well as incompetent nursing practices professional conduct, discipline as well as formal complaints and grievance procedures, students' medical requirements as well as chemical impairment for nurses in the classroom and the nursing simulation lab as well as clinical practice guidelines and guidelines, to name a few. The handbook also serves as the primary source of information on actions that fall outside the nurse's area of practice in addition to the college's guidelines and forms for clinical incidents.

The handbook for students isn't an ordinary document you get upon gaining admission into university. There's more to it than the basic information. It'll inform you of the different procedures and guidelines that the school follows and will keep you informed about the school's calendar in addition. It will also inform you of the prerequisites of the program in relation to internships, assignments, or externships as well as internships. Additionally, you'll need to be aware of the official website of your institution to ensure that you aren't missing anything that is not found in the handbook.

Additionally, since the site is regularly changed, it's going to serve as the main source of information about campus for you.

HELP FROM MENTORS AND FACULTY

The topic has been discussed before. should you be in doubt regarding any problem, it is best to seek out the student services department or your academic adviser to get additional guidance regarding the issue. A student's handbook should usually offer the guidance that you are looking for. If you're looking for something else it is necessary to have the perspective of a human (i.e. or the direction of a person you can confide in). For those situations it is possible to reach out to your adviser or mentor.

Other than professors and faculty If your school has a peer mentoring program, and you've been given a peer mentor the person you're assigned to is an excellent resource for knowledge. If you want to talk to your peer mentor to raise concerns with regard to an assignment, a particular requirement or specific processes. The information on grants and scholarships and guidance regarding how to apply for them is essential, as well as the mentor will provide useful information as well as inform you of different deadlines. Stay connected while you're in school. This can make a difference between a successful graduation or one that is a mess of missed chances.

Chapter 8: Methods of Organization

While in nursing school, students are expected to complete a variety of assignments and assignments. There is no guarantee that instructors to notify that you of the due date for something. It is necessary to manage multiple activities simultaneously as well as meeting deadlines for multiple projects, and concentrating on various demands. The ability to organize is among the best skills you can acquire, which can not only assist you achieve your goal but also make you successful in the field of nursing. It is essential to organize yourself! Begin to organize before the start of classes and keep this routine through the entire semester. It is all you need to do so you'll be able to get through the chaos and confusion in nursing school.

WAYS TO STAY ORGANIZED IN NURSING SCHOOL

We'll now take a look at some most basic methods to remain at a steady pace in nursing school We've already covered some of these in Chapter 2. have covered in Chapter 2.

Use a daily planner or calendar to record the assignments, tasks and class schedules. Complete the calendar by the start of your semester. So you'll have a clear idea of what to expect from the weeks to come. It's much simpler to arrange all of your activities around school, and it's much more efficient rather than waiting till the very last minute to finish tasks and assignments, and also to study to take tests.

Create a designated room in your home exclusively for studying or doing the nursing school work.

Use different color notebooks for different classes.

Participate in an study group along with competent nursing students from the classes you are in. Your group members must be people you are at ease with.

Create a network of mentors and nurse buddies to help your.

File loose documents that you may possess. The papers should be organized with Post-its.

Use handy supplies like Post-its. They can be used for notes that you can write to yourself, and then quickly recall the function each piece of paper serves. This can save you lots of time.

Make a study plan prior to any exam.

Notes should be written clearly or make an outline for particularly difficult subjects.

You should have many different highlighters. These can be used for marking the crucial sections in your textbooks as well with your notes as well as to select different shades for various kinds of categories.

Allocate a specific duration of time to exercise. workout.

Plan time with families and your friends too. It is just as important to relax when study, so you must be taking a mental break each month. Plan something fun like a trip to the cinema, going bowling, or taking a trip for dinner.

GETTING ORGANIZED FOR CLINICAL

Clinicals are a crucial part that are part of the nursing program. They are a brand completely new experience when you first begin your nursing education because they're very distinct from the usual courses in theory. Be prepared for them prior to the start and deal with the subject in a systematic manner. It's important to design an outline of the sheet and write down the entire information in a neat and organized method. Below are some tips that can help you keep well-organized in your clinical work:

1. Be sure to get your demographics correct Include the name of your patient and room's identifier, along with other details such as gender, age admission date and weight, height as well as allergies.

2. The patient must have an admissions diagnosis, as well as any prior medical records, as well as any surgical records.

3. There is also data on your diet and exercise degree.

4. It is possible to have a tiny box on the other side for the vital signs. It is possible to note the important information in columns. After this, you can check the box when you've charted the vitals.

5. Make a separate section to include treatment and medication. It is the place provide the necessary details like when an application of a dressing to a wound must be applied or what supplies will be required.

This is a simple sheet should be kept basic so that you are able to quickly refer to it frequently. A lot of complexity can destroy things, making information unorganized. This sheet will ensure that you don't need to waste trying to find the right place to put down your information or follow the flow of your reports. It is possible to tailor the report to suit your needs and preferences.

THE ESSENTIAL SKILL OF TIME MANAGEMENT

An overwhelming workload puts an immense strain on your time. Nursing school puts a lot of demands on your time.

To be successful in the school it is necessary to handle the vital resource of time in a smart and efficient manner. Alongside managing your time, organization is essential to success in the environment of nursing school as you'll have many things to accomplish, and just a small period of time to accomplish this.

The National Student Nurses' Association affirms that there are many elements that nurses must be able to master if they wish to excel in their career. They need to have:

Academic capability to be able to pass all subject areas.

A thirst for knowledge

A compassionate and understanding attitude

Confidence and determination to make a profession of nursing

A strong feeling of responsibility for the profession they have chosen

Proper time-management skills

It could be the most important crucial factor, according to the organization Time management, however it is the top concern for nurses, and they must incorporate the subject into their curriculum. This is that college counselors and faculties of nursing constantly develop time management strategies that help nursing students cope with the demands of their nursing studies.

The counselors frequently remind students to follow a program that doesn't compromise their chance of successfully completing the curriculum. The only thing you should do is stick to the timetable you've created. If, at any time, in the course of your plan, it's best to fill in any time you can to avoid delays in other tasks.

HAZARDS OF TIME CONSTRAINTS--A NURSE SHORTAGE

Problems with time management force nurses to transfer to different baccalaureate-level courses because they are struggling to cope with the demands and workload of the curriculum. The students find it difficult to handle the demands on their time which the course imposes.

Many factors impact the number of nurses, however at the time there are a lot of nursing students. The fewer nurses exist, the less likelihood that healthcare facilities will expand. That is why it is crucial for nurses to master the art of time management to ensure they can finish the course and then become certified nurses.

EFFECTIVE TIME-MANAGEMENT SKILLS

In order to manage your time efficiently it is essential to follow the guidelines below.

You must be organized and organize the activities you do according to your priorities. Utilize time-saving tools like appointments and calendars, and files to the track of all your tasks. A well-organized workplace can help greatly with using your time effectively.

Create a realistic schedule. administration plans out the timetables for study and duties during the first week of term. Make your other schedules in line with. Setting a realistic timetable helps you to complete all the required programs but without delaying other things.

Be aware that nursing is a high-risk degree program. Do not overburden yourself. Take breaks that last at least 10 to 15 minutes in the middle of your class tasks. This can help you relax.

Practice effective study techniques--
Consider the nursing class as a war and
make sure you have your arsenal at hand
by being prepared to take any exam that is
not announced as well as recitals. Develop
effective study habits.

Always be prepared for unexpected
situations. If you get unwell, you should be
able to adjust your schedule to
accommodate.

If you implement these time-management
techniques and methods in your daily
schedule, you'll never regret choosing a
nursing school.

Chapter 9: Goal Setting

For a successful college experience, you have established goals in both the short and long term. They're essential for your education at college. If you don't have these objectives you will not have the direction and focus. In the case of someone looking to pursue a degree within a particular area, having a defined objective helps them determine whether their graduate or baccalaureate-level education will be in line with their career objectives. In the end, define your objectives, keep them in mind!

MACRO- AND MICRO-LEVEL GOALS

Like we said earlier You can organize your course by breaking it into manageable pieces as well as setting small objectives to achieve towards larger dates. These are the micro-level objectives of your nursing program. These goals are going to prepare you to take on bigger challenges as time passes and will eventually determine the future of your career. These goals will eventually give way to macro-level, long-term goals for career development that are beyond your nursing degree.

Re-evaluate your objectives for your career, both in the immediate as well as long-term to decide the appropriate level and kind of nursing training that's necessary for you to reach the goals. It is important to consider what you'd like to accomplish in 5 to 10 years' time. This is your goal at a macro level that can help you determine your professional and personal future.

SHORT-TERM GOALS AND THEIR SIGNIFICANCE

It is common for people to mistake goals for long-term strategies and aren't aware of the importance of goals that are short-term. Goals of every nursing student is based upon the development of his or her career throughout his or her professional profession, beginning with the acceptance into the nursing school. Class-by-class, chapter-by-chapter, semester-by-semester, and treatment-by-treatment, nursing students must set small, short-term goals, to achieve the longer-term goal of graduating from the nursing program and attaining a tenured nursing occupation. When the milestones in their career progress and goals are set, they will become increasingly ambitious.

Any kind of goal is important in keeping nurses focussed on providing top-quality service and attentiveness, with care specifically for patients who require sensitive treatment and implementing the techniques and protocols that they have learned regularly, as well as to each patient. A focus on goals helps nurses stay an awareness of the most important aspects including managing time and other related concerns in the course of their job and managing education materials.

PLANNING FOR THE CAREER AHEAD

Goals for the long term are equally important. It's important to keep the fact that being ambitious can be a good thing. Aims like a reduced time-to-work, a higher pay or an easier environment for nurses are not uncommon. Thus, any nursing student must always keep a hospital in the forefront. Beginning the conversation with this institution at an early stage will speed up the process towards achieving his objectives. Managements have a negative view of nurses with qualifications who show little interest in advancing their expertise and moving forward.

Talk about your future career goals with your counselor at the nursing program you're in, or with nurses working within roles you are interested in, or even with other nurses with a similar age in your college. It's also possible to talk with graduates who just finished their degree.

Sharing your professional and personal nursing goals will help improve your interpersonal and social abilities as well as aid in the development of your skills in patient-care settings. In particular, nurses of hospitals, who manage the staff, are keen in nurses that can perform and analyze all lab outcomes related to a specific area of nursing.

Keep in mind that the objectives of nurses tend to shift as is moving from one step into the next. Nurses in the student phase are more focused on the chapter's next test, or the final test of their course in addition to a being able to graduate into more advanced classes in nursing.

Chapter 10: Reading and Writing Skills

Reading is a crucial aspect of learning. It aids in the retention of the information you've learned. It also assists you in remembering information for longer durations. Making a habit out of studying all material can greatly help you when it comes to nursing college. It is possible that you could have sailed through high school using only notes from class or Cliff Notes However, this isn't at all in college especially in the rigorous course in nursing schools.

If you're in nursing school and you're hoping to get through the long and rigorous program it is necessary to develop the practice of at the very least, studying all of the texts that are part of the program. This is only the most basic requirement to be able to do well academically. This isn't an easy task however, it's not impossible either. You just need dedication and focus.

IMPORTANCE OF READING IN NURSING SCHOOL

At nursing schools Reading is the most effective way to follow the curriculum as well as keeping track of the content being taught in the class. The most effective way to tackle the required readings is to be attentive to the course outline and then read relevant material prior to the class. By doing this, it will not only help you to be more prepared, but you will also be more successful in comparison to other students. You'll be able to comprehend the ideas as well as the topics that will be covered during the class. Reading can also provide additional benefits. If you stumble across an article or topic in a task that you are unable to comprehend You can make notes and ask the instructor to clarify it in the class. You will not only solve your questions effectively and in a efficient manner and you'll be able to be a part of the class more actively and active. The research has proven that we generally pay attention more to classes when we're already familiar with what is the instructor is teaching, in contrast to learning about topics in the first place.

DON'T UNDERESTIMATE ASSIGNED AND SUGGESTED READING

Any trick that can help you be successful or survive at nursing school will tell the same thing: complete the reading materials (both the material that is required and the ones that are advised). It should help you understand how crucial reading is in the nursing program. Make sure you follow the syllabus of your instructor that details the suggested and required studying material. Do not skip reading chapters, or the case that you're in a shortage, complete the course afterward. It is important to note down any issues that you may encounter while doing the studies, and in the event that you have to you should ask your instructor during class or at the end of the lecture for clarification. If you don't answer any questions that you be able to ask about the course or subject will affect your marks and leave you with an opportunity to grow. We've discussed it before it's not just about the grades. The focus is on learning the skills that may help save lives in the future. If you're a nurse who is passionate then you'll know how crucial reading is.

IMPORTANCE OF WRITING SKILLS IN NURSING

Writing is essential to nursing, for many reasons. Care for patients, concerns about nursing responsibility, along with a myriad of other nursing abilities all depend heavily on writing as a method as well as a method of communication. Nurses compose their notes, performing research on patients as well as conducting scholarly research.

Many experts say that the most important thing for undergraduate students training, especially for programs that are medically focused will be to help students in becoming fluent writing and spoken language. This underscores the significance of the writing ability for nurses. Nurse educators must develop educational methods to make sure that requirements of the workplace for accountability are easily measured and that they are 100% accurate fair, trustworthy, and reasonable. Many consider that in the nursing profession the predominant tendency to exchange information via oral means results in a dismissal of the value of writing in the nursing profession.

Writing for nursing students does not just improve their writing skills, but it also aids in knowledge and critical thinking. Research suggests that those who have negative feelings to assignments to write, it's typically due to a lack of support and resources to conduct research. Conscientizing that better communication skills enhance the effectiveness for effective nursing care Colleges have set up facilities, such as writing labs that help students develop favorable attitudes towards researching and writing.

HOW TO DEVELOP WRITING SKILLS

Writing is an essential component of the communication skills required to establish professional nursing methods. It is essential to be able to write clarity, precision logic, rational, and proper presentation of opinions, thoughts as well as values within nursing to ensure quality services to patients, families and the communities. To be proficient at writing communication, nursing students must continually improve their analytical, technical and persuasion skills.

If you are unsure of their writing capabilities you have the possibility of enrolling into a beginner's composition course. Additionally, there are internet-based sources. They can assist students in nursing improve their or her writing abilities.

Chapter 11: Managing Social Life

People who say the college experience is about studying, not socializing with fellow students or socializing do not understand how important socializing and networking in the current modern, connected and fast-paced society. Socializing and making connections is as important as a component of the college life as the study. Many argue that it's a vital life skill the present day. It is essential to be involved with your social activities in college. This doesn't mean you should join fraternities, or party all night at events. There's a right as well as the wrong way to approach everything but moderation is the crucial factor in this case. Learn how to manage your social schedule with the studies.

CREATING YOUR VERY OWN PROFESSIONAL NETWORK

The development to the Internet and social media websites have indeed transformed the world into a tiny area. The internet has made it easier for people to connect than they did in the past. Consider this: a lot of us remain connected to more than half the people that we were in the high school of, even though it's only through Facebook and Twitter. It was different just a few years back. Social media today plays an essential role in capable of establishing and maintaining professional relationships that extend beyond the academic setting.

As you begin the college system, you make friendships and establish many bonds. The majority of these relationships won't last past campus time and gradually disappear after graduation. There are many friends you'll keep in touch to even when the course is over. It could be friends from your room, members of the study groups, great classmates as well as professors. It will be the start of your professional circle when you begin your journey into the world of work. These individuals are in the early stages of their careers just as that you are. However, it is important to remember the fact that, like you they'll soon progress to higher levels and could be in positions of power at some point. There is no way to know if the connections you make will prove useful in the future. professional career. Maintaining meaningful relationships that go beyond university period.

Websites such as LinkedIn and Tagged make the job of professional networking easy and easy. In the past, few knew about the concept and even less understood the importance of it, however today keeping in touch is valued as a top priority. In your nursing professional career and beyond, it is imperative to keep connected to your peers in your field along with specialists from other areas of medical. It will help you stay informed about current events in your job and utilize all the tools available for advancement. Your network plays a major role in bringing you into contact with various professionals within the field.

CREATE YOUR SUPPORT NETWORK

The stressful environment and heavy work load of nursing school is often stressful for the individual, and in some cases overburden you. However, there are a variety of methods to relax, let go of the stress and release any negative energy. Be aware that all your efforts are in vain if you put everything on you. Humans are social animals, and are always in need of companionship regardless of the kind of person someone might seem. Humans are made to be social creatures. There are times of quiet, where we reflect and contemplate. There is however a major different between solitude and loneliness. You want first, and not latter.

No matter how sad or happy there is always somebody to talk to. It's always a good idea to have a friend around particularly in the nursing program, it is best to avoid going by yourself. In nursing school, you will face immense amounts of pressure academically that can be found in exams, tests, exam questions, projects, clinical experience and so on. There will be people whom you take on this load.

FRIENDS VERSUS FACEBOOK FRIENDS

The world has become technologically driven that we're frequently evaluated based on the social aspects like the amount of Facebook friends we've got. If we have more people on our list of friends, more socially accepted as we believe. Therefore, it is of immense importance for us. When we meet someone new and we want to add them to our list of friends in Facebook. Once you graduate from university and start interacting with strangers, you'll notice that your Facebook buddies are growing by just a couple hundred. Let me share one tip Five meaningful, intimate family members will have a greater value than five hundred Facebook buddies have no idea about.

When you're in college, it's important to have people you can count on. People who are not just possible contacts in the professional world. If you ever need to vent, grieve, or just squeal in joy it's likely that you'll realize the college experience much easier and, certainly enjoyable, if there's someone you can turn to in more than an acquaintance in a professional way. In many cases, we make relationships in the college setting that are likely to last for a long time.

STAY CONNECTED WITH FAMILY

If a student is leaving the comforts of home and family for first time, it is a very difficult change, and often depression and feelings of loneliness can develop. Be prepared to combat these thoughts. It is always helpful to keep in contact to family members via email or phone. Or better, using social media platforms that allow video chats. Technology has made staying communicating with family members significantly easier and more convenient than ever. When you are able to communicate frequently with your family It will be more easy to remain positive and quicker to adjust the changing environment. This typically takes a while and can be a slow process.

MASTER YOUR FINANCES

For many students, the college experience is the first time they'll be without their family. This is a completely new thing that many students be able to handle everything on their own. From shopping for groceries to school and everything that students have to be able to manage their own needs in a completely different setting. One thing that's possibly the most important aspect for living on your own is managing the finances. If a student is enrolled in college they has to pay particular attention to costs. It is due to two factors. As we have experienced, if expenses are not controlled the cost of living tends to increase quicker than the speed of a tsunami. Furthermore, a lot of young people have no experience, or are in a state of confusion, on the best way to manage costs. Most students face difficulties with money begin as soon as they're accepted to colleges, as most schools offer extremely expensive fees which require one form of financial aid.

THE FINANCIAL AID FACTOR

The cost the cost of a child's education is an important occasion. In certain cases this amount is equivalent to the price of buying a house. The cost of college is rising in America It is not surprising that parents view their capacity to cover these expenses with just a little anxiety. The abundance in financial assistance has helped make the process somewhat simpler. One of the first things you need to determine if you need financial assistance or otherwise. Many colleges offer grants and loans for certain students chosen based on their performance in competitive tests. These scholarships and grants will save you plenty of hassles. The best option is to take these tests, since it could save your family some cash. Alongside merit-based scholarships, a majority of college-bound students are eligible for a form of financial aid that is based on needs and also. The federal government is actually, the most significant source of this aid. It is easy to conduct an Internet search and find many scholarships in the subject you are studying.

MANAGING EXPENSES IN COLLEGE

The ability to manage money can not only help students well at college but throughout the remainder of your existence. There will always be a need to control your money, which includes savings and investment. Think of college as an introduction into the field of finance management. If you are able to master it effectively during college and graduate with the ability be beneficial for the remainder of your life. The first step to record is to sketch the essential expenses as well as other expenses that you will incur during your time at the college. Next, create your own budget to aid in determining the amount you'll need to cover expenses, and the amount you want to set aside for leisure pursuits. Make sure to save an amount for emergencies.

Include within your budget are the costs for food, books expenses, entertainment, and bills. It is important to not just creating an amount, but adhering to the plan. The budget you choose should be crafted in accordance with your requirements and flexible enough to adjust, should it be necessary.

THE PARTY FACTOR

Life in college has been a time of partying and having enjoyable times. It is also the time that the majority of young people step away from their homes for the first time, ready to go on a journey away from home in their own way, according to their own way. Many feel that it is the perfect time to the plunge into new experiences and let loose. Yet, don't forget that the actions you take right now, and the way you go about these important year, will decide the course and form of your professional career. Have fun and have a good time, but be careful not to harm the health of your study or yourself. This is an important balance you'll have to figure out yourself and adhere to a strict regimen if you want to be successful in any educational setting even the nursing school.

Everyone should take time out to relax and have a chat, particularly with such a busy setting and with such an overwhelming work load. Everybody needs a break every now and then. However, that's what you should expect from a party at college, a moment of relaxation. Do not make it a part of living.

Chapter 12: Open Minds and Internships

There are always students that enter college with the exact field they'd like to pursue a degree in. But there are others who have no notion of their goals for the future. A different group does have a good understanding of their career objectives, but are not sure of the fields to help them achieve these targets. But, most students end up finding themselves changing fields of study at one point in the course of their college. As an example, once you enter college, you might have a predetermined perspective that is based on a specific group of concepts. It is possible that we believe these ideas can help us reach our desired goal. However, when we experience various new experiences, and interact with many more people we are prone to change our mindsets and discover what our real desires or goals and dreams are. It causes us to alter our direction. take our lives. That's for the majority of students who go to nursing schools change majors midway through their program. It is therefore essential to remain open about your academics, and also to find out more about your interests in academics as well as your passions. At this time, you should consider options for how your passions could lead to a profession.

KEEP AN OPEN MIND

We have discussed that many students begin college with precisely what they intend to accomplish in their lives but they still take a 180 degree turn halfway throughout the course. It is possible in the event that you begin your college with an open-minded mind and are open to anything you encounter. This is the only way to uncover or strengthen your interests and interests and turn them into an effective job. If you keep a fixed way of life, not exploring different subjects, you risk staying with something which you initially enjoyed but then became bored with afterward. If you don't try something different and you'll never be able to tell if it's a good fit for you or perhaps not! Therefore, don't be afraid to try new things.

CHOOSE THE MAJOR

While you consider the college that is the best for you Be aware that uncertainty is expected. It's a process to select the right major could be thrilling. Keep in mind that you're not the only one in your situation. will have the assistance of advisers from the academic and peer departments.

The term "major" simply refers to an area of study that students may focus on. For most schools, about one third and half of your courses belong to your particular field or closely related to the subject. For most colleges that are four years are only required to choose a major close to the close the second semester of your senior year. In order to prepare, enroll in courses that appeal to you or a topic that inspires you. Be sure to are interested in the subject matter, however. It's always easier to succeed in class if you're passionate about it as well. Your enthusiasm will be maintained throughout college as well as into the professional world. The subject you select is likely to determine your future work, and also.

BROADEN YOUR HORIZONS

The college experience shouldn't focus on only academics and graduation. There are many aspects other than just the grades, homework, or the internships. College is a place where you intend to work as a nurse which should be the primary goal. Additionally, you must have the confidence to try different things beyond the classroom. It will allow you to build your character while at the college. Personal growth is an essential aspect of a college experience as there are plenty of chances to grow your life. It should be a complete learning experience that is it should not be limited only to the classes.

Based on what interests you depending on your interests, there are numerous options for activities or join clubs you could join. All it comes down to the choices you make and your interests. In the case of example, you could be a member of a club for students or run for the student administration, or even try your hand on a team of sports at your school. There are some colleges that offer cheap travel options and excursions. These types of opportunities are sure to enrich your college experience as well as give you a break from the stress of studying.

ACTIVITIES GALORE

Certain colleges offer studies abroad programmes. They are a fantastic way to explore new locations as well as cultures, while learning about the ways that nursing is different across the globe. Your mentor or college advisor will be able to provide additional information on this as well as identifying financing choices.

Each year, college campuses across all over the world organize extracurricular events through clubs and associations for students. There are clubs that you can join that shares your interests or just take part in various activities and activities without signing up for a club in case your schedule does not permit it. It is also possible to participate in intercollegiate contests as well as exhibitions and communities development initiatives which are run by nearly all nursing schools every year. A lot of colleges host famous guest lecturers as well as volunteering opportunities within the area in which they're located.

Sports are everywhere. Every college is home to one type of team. These range from baseball, volleyball, football, softball and basketball, to sports for individuals such as tennis or swimming. There are facilities at colleges for major indoor sports, such as chess, table tennis or wrestling. It doesn't matter if you are skilled in a particular game to be able to play the game. The majority of colleges provide sporting and athletic facilities for students who want to have fun. In fact, hostels also offer these amenities and facilities for the use of students. There are two choices to take part in a team, and then play the sport at a competitive stage in the intercollegiate circuit as well as take advantage of sports to relax between the intense studying. Keep in mind that these sports serve as a supplement to learning and study and should not infringe on time that you could otherwise dedicate to your studies.

THE INTERNSHIP

An internship experience is considered to be one of the crucial aspects of any medical program Nursing is not other. The nursing schools will recommend students pursue an internship. A job is more extensive and detailed than an externship that can be highly monitored and is only short-term. The internship provides the trainee with a the chance to test their skills within the field of work, as well as to see how the system works. This will allow the student to determine whether you'll be a good fit for the position as well as add knowledge on your resume.

THE STUDENT NURSE INTERNSHIP PROGRAM

The majority of hospitals and clinics have an intern program for students offered to nursing students. It's an "earn-while-you-learn" program that's designed to facilitate the transition from student to practicing nurse. The program lets students learn in a workplace and enhance their knowledge prior to their graduation.

The objectives of any significant nursing program is to:

Give the intern an the opportunity to show that they understand and ability to master technical skills and procedures that are related to the area in which they specialize.

Give the trainee with an chance to use clinical judgement and analytical thinking abilities in the process of nursing especially in the administration of care for patients.

Develop intern's abilities to manage their time and make decisions.

Provide an orientation to an intern on their specialization unit at the clinic or hospital.

The majority of hospitals and clinics offer an internship program in these fields:

Medical-Surgical

Intensive Care

Progressive Care

Perioperative

Emergency Room

Neonatal Intensive Care (NICU)

Obstetrics

Pediatrics

LPN

Open Heart Intensive Care

Applying to intern in the majority of hospitals is fairly easy. In most cases, you do not have to visit the establishment for yourself. It is easy to go on the website of the institution and submit your application on the internet. A typical nursing job is only a couple of weeks in length, however there's no set length of time. The length of the course is dependent on the specific hospital as well as regions. It can also vary with different internship programs at one hospital.

Some of these internships include a stipend in addition. In general, the salary can be anywhere from $20 to $25 per hour. This includes advantages. In order to qualify it is necessary to present an official statement of your eligibility to be able to take the NCLEX of the relevant State Board of Nursing. If you don't possess the certification of eligibility can nevertheless have an opportunity to work, however it may not be an opportunity to earn money.

Chapter 13: Victory over Obstacles

In the course of nursing it is common to encounter interruptions of one kind or the other. Most of the time, these distractions divert our attention away from the main responsibilities of the curriculum and lead us to focus on different issues. The most notable example is when you're facing the challenge of completing specific general education courses which may not be relevant to nursing, yet must be completed to earn the degree you need. Many nursing students are frustrated as they think they are wasting their time and energy is wasted on the focus on trivial things. They think that they could efficiently use their time doing things that are "productive" that is more connected to their profession. It can manifest as a feeling of discontent and can lead to feeling alienated to the student.

In this moment the focus should be on your options and realize that the program could not be as important to the field you imagine. Although some courses may seem irrelevant to nursing, you should keep your mind in the present that you need to complete them in order to realize your goal of becoming an nurse. The disappointments or negative emotions which you feel hinder your progress. The only way to overcome the obstacles is to confront them face-to-face and win.

I've said it before I've said it before, and I'll repeat that once more: the nursing program isn't a walk through the woods. The challenge of tackling and surviving the rigorous nursing curriculum isn't an easy task for a kid. It's arduous, demanding thorough, demanding determination, focus and perseverance. However, if you're dedicated to nursing, every challenge will be used as a motivation, and not a hurdle. You'll find each challenge invigorating--inspiring you to do better and better each time. Be positive regardless of the obstacles you'll encounter throughout the course.

It is crucial to stay focused at the goal. There are times the work load can be daunting, and you'll find yourself feeling lost and confused. That's when you need to be able to step back and reflect on what is the most crucial thing most people forget that is why you opted to pursue a career in nursing at all in the first place. If you're truly committed to this profession and think of the profession as more than just a means of achieving achieve a goal and you'll get an answer quickly. You'll be aware that you wish to work as a nurse so that you can assist people, help patients overcome their suffering and suffering, and make sure that they are healthy and happy of those who cannot take care of themselves.

If you've got the information in your head and you've got your sights set at the end of the tunnel and your vision, you'll see that no challenge is large enough to cause you to wander away from your path. Your determination should be more powerful than any challenges you encounter.

Chapter 14: decided to become a Nurse

There are many people who are unsure on how to apply into nursing schools, what is the best school for them, and also what is the real experience. Students who are also juggling other obligations including a job, and an extended family, may be wondering if they can manage the pressures of college and work. When you begin to think about what you can do to manage everything, you have decide the best way to begin this journey.

Which Is The Right Program For Me?

The most common question individuals ask is "Where should I go?" It may be an obvious concern for the majority of people, however for some individuals, the answer could seem difficult to answer. There are various kinds of courses that are available each with its specific requirements to be admitted This article will detail the distinctions of each to help those who are interested. First, you should ask yourself is which qualification you'd like to pursue, and take your choice from the answers. Nurse programs within the U.S. can provide you with a diploma, associate's degree, and even a bachelor's degree even if you already hold an education in another area. A few nurses decide to pursue an associate's degree initially, after which they return for school to earn their bachelor's degrees with the help of the employer. Whatever path you choose to follow, the most appropriate one for you will be the one that leads you the RN with your name!

Nursing is among the handful of professions that allow you to remain employed as a nurse with any formal education. However, it's not as prevalent as it once was. This is due to a period where hospitals required nurses however there was no program that taught nurses the necessary skills for their job. Therefore, hospitals began programs to train these nurses, and provide the nurses with diplomas upon completion of their course, which acknowledged they'd completed all the requirements to become an effective nurse. Hospitals liked the program since the students offered work for free, and nurses appreciated the course however the program was more of a practice-based experience, and contained no nursing theories.

There were tens of thousands of these programmes all over the nation. In the present, there are just less than 100 of them operating. One of the best ways to discover the existence of an accredited diploma program in your area (besides Google!) is to reach out to the State's Board of Nursing and ask. One of the advantages of enrolling in one of these programmes is that you'll likely gain more actual nursing work as opposed to if were enrolled in a bachelor's or associate's degree program. a bachelor's program. It is possible to take the exact NCLEX certification exam as nursing graduates from a bachelor's or associate's degree course takes. The drawback of these types of courses is that some hospitals pay nurses according to the level of level of education they've received and, if you don't have a qualification, you could be lower wages for doing similar work to those who have degrees.

Associate degrees are a well-liked option for aspiring nurses. It typically takes approximately two to three years be completed at a community college offering a great mix of education in science in addition to nursing theories and practical instruction. It is common to complete them in part-time, during the night or over weekends, giving the possibility of students who are juggling more responsibilities like a work or a family to take care of. A majority of associate degree programs cost less than a bachelor's program in a four-year institution which makes them a desirable alternative for those worried about funding their educational expenses. When they graduate, nurses who hold an associate's diploma can take the same test as nurses with a bachelor's diploma are required to pass. However, the disadvantage of not being able to pass having an associate's diploma is that a few hospitals possess been seeking to obtain the designation "Magnet" status. This award is given to hospitals by the American Nurses' Credentialing Center to those hospitals that meet a set of standards that are designed to assess the quality and the quality of the nursing staff they employ. One of these criteria is that all nurses on the personnel have a bachelor's degree or higher in the field of education and that is why it's impossible for nurses who have an associate's degree not being qualified to be employed.

The bachelor's level of nursing is the most common route to earn this degree. Bachelor's degrees are obtained in just four years of study at an institution like a university or college. The students can begin their studies straight from high school, or be returning after gaining experience in their lives. Each school's curriculum is unique the majority of schools demand approximately half of the credits to be earned in general education subjects, like mathematics, English as well as science, and the history of science. About a quarter of these credits is usually determined by the student's discretion and may be a part of extracurricular subjects that are of interest (Wildflowers from Nevada for instance?) or as a minor subject. About a quarter of the credits awarded are within the major area of study that for a nurse student will be nursing and associated courses. Benefits of earning an undergraduate diploma for nursing is the fact that it typically is accompanied by a higher amount of salary than nurses with degrees that are associate's. However, the additional cost for four years in university can mean that some of your extra earnings will go towards paying off the student loan in the first place!

If you've already completed an undergraduate degree from another area, but are thinking of nursing as a possible second career and a second degree program might be ideal for those who are interested! These kinds of programs take into account the courses you have already taken prior to obtaining the first degree. They they are designed to teach students about the field of nursing. There are some programs that can be completed in as short as a year. Additionally, they offer flexible choices that permit students to take classes at night, on during weekends, or even via online. It's a great alternative to re-enter an occupation that you could find yourself unhappy with. A caveat however is that if it's longer than 10 years since your last time at college, you might need to complete some of the required courses. One of the disadvantages of programs such as those are that a lot of colleges offer scholarships to those who are in pursuit of their first degree. As such, they may have less funds accessible and you could need to borrow additional loans. Some one-year programs will restrict you from working when you're in the course. Therefore, it is important to prepare financially and emotionally for that kind of change in your life.

When you've settled on the kind of degree you'd like to pursue begin looking into the various schools offering that degree. You should ask yourself whether you prefer to keep your house close and if you'd like to travel across the country to experience a change in scenery or the pace. Look through every school's site for a better understanding of how their programs work. Join various communities and forums and engage with the students that are there to find out what they enjoy and dislike about their school. When I was searching I discovered that allnurses.com is a fantastic way to meet other students and potential students as well as gather information on a particular school. Don't end there! Make contact with the school and speak to admissions officials. The school will usually host Open Houses on campus where visitors can tour the campus to see labs and classrooms. You can also organize for one-on-one visits that allow you to inquire about the college and the programs they have to offer.

Wisdom pearls:

If you meet an admissions representative, either during the Open House or at a one-on-one interview be sure to give them a thanks note following the meeting! The note doesn't need to be elaborate, it's simply a couple of lines on how much you liked visiting the school and how you hope to visit in the future as an undergraduate.

As I considered attending nursing schools I set up an Excel spreadsheet in my laptop with the various schools I was thinking I would like to apply to. I wrote the name of the schools on first, then on the bottom, I wrote down details I needed to find out. This included for me essential information like how much each school would cost as well as how far it was from the school to my home, as well as the diverse prerequisites each program required to be able to enroll admitted. Was I required to pass an exam? Write an essay? When was the deadline for applications? I took notes on it all. I listed nursing school courses which I believed I would be able to get towards, and ones I thought I could get into. When I was done with my list, I started formulating my strategies. I understood what I was required to accomplish, as well as the date I needed to finish it before the deadline. The Resources section on the rear of this book is an example of the spreadsheet that I used.

What About Testing?

There are some exams you may need to pass to be admitted to the nursing college that you prefer. This includes tests like the TEAS test, SAT or ACT or the GRE. It's good to know that you don't need to be able to pass the tests all at once! But the downside is that you'll probably need to complete at least one of them to qualify for the nursing school of your dreams.

The TEAS test stands for the Test of Essential Academic Skill it is an element of admissions procedures by hospitals and nursing schools all over the world. The test is a standardised way to assess the ability of a person in several crucial areas. It is designed to determine students who can achieve success in nursing school as well as are able to be nurses. The test is divided into four parts which take about four hours to finish. Reading section comprises 40-question and requires fifty minutes to finish the test. Charts, paragraphs, passages or graphs are all acceptable to aid in the process, with the aim to assess your ability to identify important elements within the texts. The section on math runs for 56 minutes it covers topics like the conversion of fractions and convert them into mathematical equations, ratios and proportions. Science has 30 topics and 38 minutes for the task. The topics may range between basic physical concepts and general science, the thing is being assessed this is your capacity to be able to think critically and not just the ability to recall information. The last section concerns English and Language usage. It comprises 55 questions that have to be completed in just 65 minutes. The section includes questions on grammar, punctuation as well as sentence comprehension, spelling and punctuation. If any portion of the test seems confusing or frightening to you, do not be scared! There are plenty of internet-based resources that permit students to attempt practice tests or go over the materials before taking the test. If you finally decide to take the test, you'll receive your results within just 48 days.

It is believed that the SAT tests are typically utilized by colleges with four years of education however, they can be included in some associate degree programs too. The SAT test your understanding of writing, reading and math. A majority of students will take the test during the junior or senior years in high school. Beginning in 2016 the SAT will be comprised of two obligatory sections, which will test reading and math. The writing section is now available as an optional. The exam will take 3 hours for completion, and the students who choose to add the writing portion will need the additional time of 50 minutes finish the writing section. Critical reading is comprised of three sections that are scored, and the test questions range between sentence completion and comprehension of passages. Quantitative, or the mathematics section is comprised by three sections scored which are either

143

multiple-choice or grid-in. Test participants must write down their answer on the paper given. There's a wide selection of courses and books that are available online as well as in person to assist you in preparing for these types of tests If this is the type of test you are required to take at your school.

It is a test that tests students' ability to think critically. ACT is a general-education test, which can be recognized by four year bachelor's program, as well as an exam that is multiple-choice in English mathematics, science and reading. It also has an optional writing test which tests the ability of students to think about and compose a brief essay. Since the beginning of 2015, this test will currently being made available as computer-based tests. The first part is 45 minutes long, 75-question test, which tests students' abilities in the use and aspects of English. The second part comprises a 60-question, one-hour section in maths, which tests your understanding of geometry, algebra and trigonometry for elementary students. The comprehension test comprises 40 tests that are which can be completed in only 35 minutes with four reading examples. The science reasoning final section will last for 35 minutes. 40-question test which tests students' ability to draw conclusions the meaning of 14 different sections. The preparation for the test could be done online, or in a class as well as many test prep solutions accessible.

The GRE stands for the Graduate Record Exam and is only required for students who already have a bachelor's degree and are applying to a nursing program that will lead to higher education, such as a bachelor's-to-master's, or bachelor's-to-doctorate program. The test is computer-driven that will assess the abilities of students in the areas of reading comprehension and critical thinking, as well as mathematical reasoning, and writing. Some cautions for returning students thinking of the test: If you took it at least 5 years ago, your results are no longer valid, and the test has to be retaken. Also when it's been longer than just a few years since the last time you were at school, then a review session is highly suggested.

How Am I Going To Pay For It All?

It's possible that you've a clear concept of the type of college you'd like to attend, and maybe you've figured out which tests you must complete to gain admission But are you thinking what you'll do to cover the cost of the whole thing? If you're not born with an empty silver spoon on your table (and many of us aren't) it is important to consider what options you have. There are several methods of obtaining the funds needed to pay for your studies. They include grants, scholarships or loans.

They are scholarships that provide free funds to students in the hopes to help them pursue the right to pursue higher education. They usually come as a one-time donation with a certain quantity, and often applicants must be a candidate for a specific scholarship. A lot of scholarships are specifically designed with an individual student for example, a person with a particular demographic of minorities or a particular location, but there are some far more specific. It's not yet found however, if you're unicycle riding, left-handed college student in Idaho you could find some scholarships available that is suitable for you too! The most effective method to locate the latest scholarships is to look them up on the internet. I suggest starting with websites such as scholarships.com, fastweb.com, and zinch.com for fun and exciting scholarships could be yours to submit an application to.

The majority of scholarships fall into two types: need-based and merit-based. These scholarships are awarded to all students, regardless of circumstances, and frequently ask to provide your grade point average. Scholarships based on need are offered where there's a clear need. Typically, you must fill out an FAFSA application to establish the eligibility criteria.

The FAFSA application sounds frightening, but really isn't. FAFSA refers to the free Application for Federal Student Aid. In order to fill out this form the application, visit fafsa.ed.gov to set up an online profile. Answer questions on how much you (and when you're sufficiently old or your parents) have earned during the preceding year. Once you have completed the questionnaire the form, you will be informed of how much your anticipated contribution to the cost of your education should be. The information you provide is passed on to the institutions you're considering or attending as well as helping them to determine the financial aid you will receive.

They are comparable as scholarships in the sense that they provide you with money and do not have to repay also. One of the most commonly used grants for schools can be the Federal Pell Grant. Federal government grants the money to those with financial needs who are not yet completing their bachelor's degree. In 2015, the maximum amount to be given is $5730 however, the amount which you get could vary based on your financial status.

Different loans are available. They are essentially borrowed money in exchange for a promise you'll return it once when you finish your degree. It is also a legal document which states exactly "I promise I will pay this money back," or the promissory note. It explains the exact amount you're borrowing, what rate of interest and the date you'll start making the repayments. There are many kinds of loans for students. the type of loan you're eligible to receive is contingent upon your individual circumstances. They can be private, federal or private. That means the company who is lending you the cash is either your federal government the state government, or even a individual with rich pockets that agrees to allow you to borrow money.

A majority of people finance their school by combining scholarships as well as loans. One of the best ways to get information about the best programs for you is to set an appointment with the school's financial aid department and talk about the matter with them. They will be able to advise you about the best options for the situation you're in, and can help you find options that you may not be aware of existed to help you.

My Application Is Asking For A Personal Statement. What Do I Do?

There are schools that have you write your personal statement. It's generally, it should read as follows "Why I want to go to Nursing School." Spend some time to think about this. Is it for admission because of an experience you had personally? Did you receive care from incredible nurses while you fell unwell? Did you care for the family member that suffered injury or illness?

Do not fret if you do not possess a compelling personal story that connects you with nursing. Perhaps your prior experiences before going to nursing school can make an impactful argument. Perhaps you've been participating in voluntary work or even research. These experiences led you to look into nursing as a career.

No matter what your subject, you must make sure you take time to write your statement. The words you write must reflect your character as a person, and your capabilities, accomplishments, aspirations and convictions. After you have completed your essay make sure you go back and read your work at least a couple of times. You can ask a friend of yours or advisor to provide opinions. If you decide to do anything, be sure you adhere to the guidelines offered by the college you're submitting your application to. Additionally, ensure that you do not make any spelling mistakes or mistakes!

Chapter 15: Classes in a lecture hall

Laboratory or in a traditional lecture hall you will have to take plenty of courses that you be required to attend when you are a nurse. Although the content of each class will vary from one school to the next however, there is a lot of commonality within each program for students in all nursing programs will be exposed to. In this section I'll discuss a selection of the classes you're likely to be taking when you are a student in nursing in addition to giving suggestions regarding the best ways to take notes and study.

What Kind Of Classes Do I Need To Take To Become A Nurse?

Wherever you go or which type of school you are enrolled in, there's likely to be several of the same courses which every nurse must complete. This includes Fundamentals of Nursing, Assessment, Pathophysiology and Pharmacology. Don't be shocked by having to study subjects such as leadership, management and informatics! The goal of the school is to help you learn to think like a nurse which is a far cry than the way you've thought throughout your entire existence. It teaches you how to analyze your needs, organize, and make the decisions you make quickly.

Nursing will teach you what must observe when a patient is experiencing decompensation, what to do in the situation along with the research regarding the reasons you'll decide to make the choices you do at that point. To be able to make this happen it is necessary to possess an extensive understanding regarding the human body. This is taught through classes such as Anatomy and Physiology in which you are taught every part of the human body as well as how they interact to allow us to be able to breathe, move or digest, which is basically the human body is competent of being alive. You will then be able to understand the human body at more of a level and understand the way that cells interact with one another in courses such as Pathophysiology. These courses are important as a fundamental knowledge of human anatomy helps you to understand the difference between what's "right" or "normal," to be able recognize unusual signs and symptoms of the patient's condition, regardless of whether they are an emergency situation or as component of their illness process. A thorough understanding of your human body's chemical makeup is essential to understand what the drugs you administer in your role as a nurse function.

The classes in Pharmacology will educate you about various types of drugs and the way they function in your body. The classes will not only teach you about different types of medicines however, you will also learn how medication is given, the way in which your body takes in the medication as well as how it breaks down and then how it's eliminated. Your teacher will explain the top negative side effects to be on the lookout for, as well as the most frequent side effects associated with the various medications. Sometimes, it can feel like you're trying to learn a different way of speaking! Yet, mastering these subjects is crucial, as you'll need this knowledge daily as a nurse at the hospital. As an nurse, you teach your patients the proper way to use their medication and also inform them about any possible side effects to inform you of. As an experienced nurse, you be aware of how the medication is designed to affect the patient. Therefore, if the medicine doesn't work and you are unable to help, consult with your patient and their doctor to alter the medication.

Courses such as Fundamentals and Assessment are going assist you to become a thinker as an experienced nurse. The classes will teach you exactly what they claim they'll cover: fundamental concepts and the way to evaluate the patient from head to the toe. Basics of Nursing will give you the fundamentals of what nursing is and how we play a contribution to life of patients. It is likely that you will be able to take a practical course to go along with your lecture and will teach you the skills needed to administer an overnight bath or to change the sheets while patients still lying in their mattress. (I'm going to go over the clinical aspects in a different section.) In Assessment in this course, you'll learn the fundamentals of evaluating your patient from head foot. The instructors will show you the symptoms of disease and health across every body system as well as learn to apply those skills to use within the clinic and also. They are great because it will be the first time you will experience the life of you are a "real" nurse!

The one thing you'll need to acquire during class that is distinct from the classes you've taken previously is writing an appropriate health plan. Care plans, in essence it is a plan to help your patient get better. There are a variety of nursing diagnosis, which differ from normal medical diagnosis which is why you should pick the diagnosis that best matches the needs of your patient. These diagnoses for nurses are known as NANDA diagnoses. Examples of them are accessible on the internet. There is the option to purchase the Nursing Diagnosis Book or a Nursing Care Plan Book that includes the diagnosis for the diagnosis itself, such as "ineffective breathing pattern," or the medical condition that includes the nursing diagnosis within (So an illness like "Pneumonia" will have "ineffective breathing pattern" identified as one of the nursing diagnosis).

If you've made the appropriate diagnosis for your patient your plan of care will include the factors that justify your diagnosis and the different strategies are used to treat the patient's condition. Care plans may differ depending upon the instruction of your institution however, the thing you're learning to accomplish is to recognize problems, understand which steps are suitable solutions for the problem and know what you should be looking for to improve the condition of the patient. These are essential skills you need to master in your job as nurses.

Wisdom pearls:

Classes in nursing can be difficult for everyone! If you feel that you're having trouble in a particular topic or idea talk to your instructor or a teaching assistant regarding the issue. You should try to improve the aspects that you are struggling with at the beginning of the term instead of having to wait until the last minute of class for you to discover that you're not sure what you need to be able to comprehend.

How Do I Take Notes? Do I Write Everything Down?

Although it might seem efficient to emphasize every phrase in your textbook, except the words "and" and "the," this isn't the most effective way to master the countless new concepts that instructors teach to you! If you're still looking for an approach that is effective for you, we've got some suggestions.

Students tend to be in two groups: those who are tech-savvy and conventional (pen as well as paper) note-taking. The category you belong to may depend on the way you learn, your experience, and your age. It is essential to choose an effective system for you, in order that you're able to learn huge amount of new knowledge and retain the latest information and blend seemingly disparate fields of study all within a just a few minutes. Although I don't recommend one kind of note-taking over another however, I will say that there's been an enormous amounts of study recently showing that students can be capable to retain more information by using pen-and-paper techniques rather than typing.

If you're a techie who wants to be paper-free the school you attend may give the students a.pdf as well as a PowerPoint version of the professor's slides before your class. Be aware, however that the notes from your teacher remain their intellectual property. They can be used to learn from, however they are not available for posting to the internet or expose them to the world. If you're using slides from the lecture then you are able to use various apps to alter them while you make notes. A few of my top applications that I use to take notes, organizing, and logging notes are Notability, Evernote and Springpad.

If you're an avid note-taking pen and paper user, you can find a couple of ways to organize your slides and notes in order. Based on my experiences I've found that there was plenty of information to keep track of that I was required take a printout of my slides prior to the lecture. If I didn't, I would be making my first draft, and the lecturer had already gone three slides forward! By having a printed copy of the slides right in front of me I was able to include the details that were discussed in the lecture, but was not visible on the slide (but frequently was in the test!). I discovered that the most efficient way to keep track of all my documents and notes was to make a separate folder for every class. There were some classmates who swear that they had a binder, which meant they printed out and punch holes in every page. They would then utilize the dividers for each class to organize their the notes. Find the best method your needs, however remain well-organized! It's not a good idea to get lost in the evening before the exam to locate the right pages from your lecture you attended just three weeks earlier.

One of the key abilities that can help to take notes for nursing school is learning how to review your notes before and after. If you're able to access the notes of your lecturer prior to the class begins, take a look and begin to gain an idea of the course will be. Note down in the margins (or the notebook) of any questions you'd like addressed. In class, if it is unclear to know what's going on and you don't understand what's being said, you will have a greater understanding of what you would like to inquire about. After class has ended, make a point to read over what you wrote as well as what was discussed. It accomplishes two goals and will not only allow you to learn the subject as well, it may aid in identifying specific areas where you'll require extra time to research further.

A few people swear by index cards. In reality I once sat in a pharmacology course with a man who sat through the whole lecture in writing down every fact on index cards when the professor was lecturing. If these cards work for you do it! Recopying the content onto cards is a fantastic option to keep the content you've read and aid you in being able to remember what you read later. If you're strapped for time or need to learn lots of material There are usually a variety of various pre-printed index cards which you can use to learn from.

Additionally, students prefer to record lectures in order to listen back to the lectures in the future. Make sure it is possible that you need either the permission of the teacher or from the institution's consent for recording lectures. As with accessing their notes, the lecture is intellectual property of the instructor. Additionally, a lot of professors don't want to publish their thoughts in social media platforms or on other websites, in order to avoid having their opinions scrutinized by people who are not part of the class. Be on the safe part and inquire.

Do I Have To Buy The Books? They Are SO Expensive!

To purchase or not buy That is the dilemma! Textbooks for colleges are frequently thought of as a fraud, because they're cost prohibitive and are often updated and make the earlier versions obsolete. The textbook issue will be addressed by the professor during the day you start class. The professor will inform you whether they're open to using the older edition (often purchased at a bargain price by a second-hand book from the bookstore at your school or through a fellow student who's taken the class) and if they think you'll require any of it. Before spending upwards of $100 for a costly dust-inducing book that aren't likely to open during the entire class, inquire with students who've taken the course prior to they. They could be able inform you if the answers to questions come directly out of the text or if your professor only uses it even once in his lectures. One option that is beginning becoming more widespread is the fact that a lot books are now available in the form of e-books. There are several benefits of this from the less expensive cost of an electronic text as well as the ability to look up the book for your subject you're researching. Remember that the library at school should contain an official textbook you will need for class. If you're not keen to purchase the book or an electronic version You can usually borrow the book from the library to study there.

Pearls Of Wisdom

Nurses employ shorthand. Many. It might be useful for you to master the shorthand to make notes more quickly and also being able to comprehend the text being written. Here's a list of some nursing shortcuts may be found in textbooks or lectures:

AC Prior to meals

Bid Twice a day

BP Blood pressure

C- - With

C/O Complaining of

D/C Discontinue or discharge

D/t Due to

F/U Follow up

Fx Fracture

HS Before bed

Chapter 16: Gaining Experience

It's very it's great to know about the theory of nursing practice. But how do you actually procedure of nursing itself? It's good news that there will be a lot of time to practice during nursing school through your clinical time. What you do with the clinical program, it will depend on the particular program you're in, however, at some time, the school will make a decision that you're able as a caregiver for an individual. In this article we'll take a examine how your experience in the clinical setting could be like and provide some tips on how to get the most the time you spend in clinical as a nurse student.

What Are Clinicals?

Your practical experiences can differ significantly based on the place the clinic is located in the particular class you're attending, however there are a lot of similarities. It is expected that you visit your clinic along with group of classmates as well as the preceptor who will teach all the information that you require to be aware of in relation to the subject at hand. The pre-conference will take place in which you'll be taught about the location as well as some of the patients you'll be taking charge of during that particular period of time. After your shift, which is typically only a couple of hours, there will be an after-conference where you can discuss the things you observed, and what you performed, and perhaps you will even present to others regarding the patient who you had to take charge of.

The ability to present a patient's story is an essential skill that can be utilized frequently during your time as a nurse. it is your responsibility learn how to communicate with the patient's condition when you turn over the care of the patient to a nurse on the following shift. Or, you'll need to talk about the treatment of the patient in hospitals during rounds. Skills you gain from post-conference training will teach how to make your presentation concise and to only focus on the aspects that another person should know, in addition to a suitable style of presentation. Most commonly, the formats for the presentation of patients is either an SBAR or SOAP note.

SBAR refers to Background, Situation Assessment and Recommendations. The situation informs another person what's happening regarding the patient. The reason for their presence? What's the problem? The Background contains all details about their past. Are they suffering from or other health conditions? Do they take any medication? The Assessment will inform to the person who is taking it that they may have to know about this specific patient. What's happening to the various systems (respiratory or cardiovascular.)? Are they able to walk? Talk? Eat themselves? Are they equipped with the Foley catheter or IV line? In the final section the report, you will provide suggestions for the treatment of their needs. What is the next step in this specific patient? Are they required to undergo further tests? Are their medicines adjusted? Do you think a different expert should be brought for consultation with the patient? It is here that you summarize everything you know about the patient, and then determine the next steps for them.

SOAP is a shorthand for Subjective assessment, Objective and Plan. It's often utilized in the process of writing notes about your patient. However, it could be utilized as a template to discuss your patient's condition with colleagues and your preceptor as well. The subjective data should include the main complaint of the patient or perhaps a short paragraph that is written by the patient explaining why they're present. Follow up by providing information regarding their background of their illness and an examination of their bodies organs. The Objective data are in which you record information on the vital indicators of your patient as well as the things you observed (or did not observe) during your assessment of the patient. The Assessment may include a variety of diagnoses of your patient's condition But remember that these are not medical diagnoses but nursing ones. medical diagnosis. If you are assessing your patient it is also recommended to include a second paragraph explaining the person who is your patient and the reason they're here. In this case, "Mr. Jones is a 37-year old man who has a background of heart disease and is in the hospital right now to have a splinter removed on his finger."

Your next step is to end with your plan, that is similar to recommendations of the SBAR report. The plan will define what your next steps and should be for the patient.

To sum up:

SBAR

Situation (what happens)

Background (what was the previous event that occurred to this patient)

Assessment (what do you observe?)

Plan (what is your plan?)

Note on SOAP

Subjective (what is the patient's story told you)

The objective (what was it that you observed)

Assessment (what did you learn regarding the subject)

Plan (what is in the next)

In your shift as a clinical nurse, it is common to be assigned an individual patient to care for or two. Although there are some laws that limit what you are not allowed to do (like administering medications to patients) but for the vast portion, you're doing your job as nurses. Learn from your teacher the correct methods regarding how you can care of the patient. This includes giving the patient a bath in bed and to change bed sheets while the patient is still asleep! Learn the proper way to place patients on bedpans as well as for more patient who is ambulatory, you'll be taught the proper methods for aiding a patient to get move off the bed in a safe manner. As you're working on your clinic and you'll learn how to use common devices in the hospital that range from heart monitors to ventilators.

If you visit your clinic site You will have the chance to get acquainted with various people who are employed in hospitals or similar care facility and get to know their duties. Be sure to inquire about how they work, as they may be able to show you important things!

Who Are The People In My Neighborhood? Some Of The Jobs At A Hospital PCAs, or Patient Care Associates. Although they might be referred to as somewhat different than the one at your facility, the roles tend to be similar from place to place. PCAs will aid you in caring for the patients that are on your floor. PCAs don't hold a license which means that you will not be able delegate the medical duties to them while you're nursing, but PCAs can help in making the lives of patients easier and more enjoyable by helping in taking care of patients' needs, such as feeding them and bathing, or even changing their clothes.

CNAs, or Certified Nursing Assistants. CNAs are certified by the state of California with the capacity to monitor vital measurements, read blood sugar readings and complete a variety of others tasks in addition to aiding in the care of demands of patients. Some hospitals have CNAs as well as PCAs perform the same duties. In the event that you're employed as a nurse maintaining a positive relationship with CNAs and PCAs within your hospital can to make your work easier and enjoyable! Make sure to show them appreciation for the hard work they perform.

Transporters aid in taking patients from location to place in the hospital. They may be able to show nurses in training how for moving a patient on the stretcher to bed without hurting your back or causing injury to your patient.

Respiratory care experts. They are highly skilled and trained to assist your patients in breathing better and could make the difference between being a happy patient or Code Blue! The members of your respiratory team will be able to teach you about the various types of oxygen-supply systems ranging from an nasal cannula to non-rebreather respirator and even devices like a ventilator, or a continuously positive airway pressure (CPAP) device.

Physical Therapists. Therapists working with patients in helping them regain or keep their mobility. They're a fantastic resource to find out how you can get the patient out safely from the bed or demonstrate how to use equipment like a walker, or Hoyer lift.

Administrative Staff. Your administrative team is the ones who must take calls from the ringing phone and transfer calls to proper nurses, and page doctors to the nursing staff when required, and occasionally oversee the huge volume of paperwork produced by your clinic. They are able to help you find who you will encounter on your shift.

Nurses. Nurses at your clinical location can be very different, for example, those who are able to meet with you and discuss with you the intricacies of their jobs and others who could have a busy schedule due to their work load and are unable to make time for a student during that particular time. Watching the nurses in action when you're on your clinic is an incredible experience, particularly when you realise that this is possible to be them in a extremely short amount of duration!

Doctors. Your doctors at your clinic facility might not have patience or time to talk to nursing students. However, they may enjoy teaching a lot. Additionally, they may be engaged in teaching medical students of their own. There's a structure among the medical professionals within your institution too particularly if your clinic location is within the context of a hospital that is a teaching facility. Understanding this hierarchy now can be beneficial when you are on your way to becoming a clinical doctor. A doctor is an intern within the first year of graduating from medical school. A resident is a medical professional who has more than a year removed from medical school but continuing to learn about their specialization. Chief residents are an individual doctor that is completing one more year of residency. They are responsible for the fellow residents. A fellow doctor is one who has finished their residency and works for the hospital with an individualized grant for some type research. A physician who is an attending physician who has completed their residency and works on their specialization within the hospital.

How Do I Prepare For Clinicals?

To conduct your clinical work it is likely that you be required to wear the uniform of your school will require for you to wear. Some schools have opted for the all-white uniform in a reference to the classic all-white uniform which nurses wore. But, it is an extremely difficult colour to maintain in good order, and certain schools have allowed students to wear various colors of scrubs. The uniform you wear will likely comprise of scrubs, footwear (usually entirely white) as well as a watch with a second-hand to allow you to monitor the pulse of your patient. Consider bringing your notebook, pen extra stethoscope, and penlight on your way to the clinic, as you'll need them frequently when you examine the patients.

A lot of nursing students would like to be aware of the white shoes required for their clinical work. There are rules that vary from one school to another However, in our school, the shoes needed to be white. That meant certain of my peers had used White-Out in order to hide any little tiny bits of color they had in their footwear! Check the rules of your school by speaking with your teachers prior to purchasing any shoes you have to paint white.

A lot of nursing students are adamant about nursing Clogs. They claim that for being at their desks for long periods at a stretch it is the best pair of shoes to choose. Yet, in the same group of the people who are enthusiastic about their footwear they also have those that are just as passionate about their shoes. For students who can't wear clogs for nursing, I recommend searching the internet for white sneakers that are comfortable and supportive. An excellent source is the websites for supply of cheerleading equipment, as the sneakers for cheerleading must be white and can withstand the rigors of a great deal of force.

A stethoscope is probably among the most expensive items you'll need in nursing school, but it's an investment that will yield great returns. Although cute the stethoscopes featuring prints and floral designs are, often hearing isn't so good. The top stethoscopes to purchase have an instrument and a bell and allow users to hear both high and low pitch sounds. Many students prefer heart stethoscopes which claim to have the highest capability to detect noises. In the end, you'll want to purchase a stethoscope is affordable and able to can hear clearly using.

There is a need for an eye-watch while working or work, as well as an additional hand. It is used to gauge the pulse of your patient when you're taking vital indicators. Personally, I love buying every rubber watch I can at the local dollar store in case something goes wrong with the watches at work, and they fail, I'm not so upset. Students and nurses who love watches that are pinned to the scrubs' front. The watch is much less likely to come into contact with patients and can aid in the control of infections.